The Ethics and Politics of Community Engagement in Global Health Research

Drawing on a growing consensus about the importance of community representation and participation for ethical research, community engagement has become a central component of scientific research, policy-making, ethical review, and technology design. The diversity of actors involved in large-scale global health research collaborations and the broader 'background conditions' of global inequality and injustice that frame the field have led some researchers, funders, and policy-makers to conclude that community engagement is nothing less than a moral imperative in global health research.

Rather than taking community engagement as a given, the contributions in this edited volume highlight how processes of community engagement are shaped by particular local histories and social and political dynamics, and by the complex social relations between different actors involved in global public health research. By interrogating the everyday politics and practices of engagement across diverse contexts, this book pushes conversations around engagement and participation beyond their conventional framings. In doing so, it raises radical questions about knowledge, power, expertise, authority, representation, inclusivity, and ethics and to makes recommendations for more transformative, inclusive, and meaningful community engagement.

This book was originally published as a special issue of the *Critical Public Health* journal.

Lindsey Reynolds is the Co-Director of the Pivot Collective in Cape Town, South Africa. She also holds honorary appointments at Brown University, Stellenbosch University, and the University of Cape Town. Her work explores the ethical and social dynamics of processes of knowledge production and circulation in global health research and implementation.

Salla Sariola is a Finnish Academy Research Fellow and an Adjunct Professor in Sociology at Helsinki University, Finland. Her work has explored the ethics and politics of science and technology, as well as gender and sexuality in South Asia and Africa. Her background encompasses science and technology studies, social study of biomedicine, and bioethics.

The Ethics and Politics of Community Engagement in Global Health Research

Edited by
Lindsey Reynolds and Salla Sariola

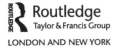

Routledge
Taylor & Francis Group

LONDON AND NEW YORK

First published in paperback 2024

First published 2020
by Routledge
4 Park Square, Milton Park, Abingdon, Oxon OX14 4RN

and by Routledge
605 Third Avenue, New York, NY 10158

Routledge is an imprint of the Taylor & Francis Group, an informa business

© 2020, 2024 Taylor & Francis

Chapter 3 © 2018 Lieke Oldenhof and Rik Wehrens. Originally published as Open Access.
Chapter 4 © 2018 Evans Gichuru, Bernadette Kombo, Noni Mumba, Salla Sariola, Eduard J. Sanders & Elise M. van der Elst. Originally published as Open Access.
Chapter 5 © 2018 Siân Aggett. Originally published as Open Access.

Publisher's Note
The publisher has gone to great lengths to ensure the quality of this reprint but points out that some imperfections in the original copies may be apparent.

Disclaimer
Every effort has been made to contact copyright holders for their permission to reprint material in this book. The publishers would be grateful to hear from any copyright holder who is not here acknowledged and will undertake to rectify any errors or omissions in future editions of this book.

British Library Cataloguing-in-Publication Data
A catalogue record for this book is available from the British Library

ISBN: 978-0-367-43777-0 (hbk)
ISBN: 978-1-03-283903-5 (pbk)
ISBN: 978-1-00-301118-7 (ebk)

DOI: 10.4324/9781003011187

Typeset in Myriad Pro
by codeMantra

Contents

Citation Information

Chapters 1–5 and 7–11 were originally published in the journal, *Critical Public Health*, volume 28, issue 3 (June 2018). Chapter 6 was published in the *Critical Public Health*, volume 28, issue 5 (September 2018). When citing this material, please use the original page numbering for each article, as follows:

Chapter 1
The ethics and politics of community engagement in global health research
Lindsey Reynolds and Salla Sariola
Critical Public Health, volume 28, issue 3 (June 2018) pp. 257–268

Chapter 2
An alternative imaginary of community engagement: state, cancer biotechnology and the ethos of primary healthcare in Cuba
Nils Graber
Critical Public Health, volume 28, issue 3 (June 2018) pp. 269–280

Chapter 3
Who is 'in' and who is 'out'? Participation of older persons in health research and the interplay between capital, habitus and field
Lieke Oldenhof and Rik Wehrens
Critical Public Health, volume 28, issue 3 (June 2018) pp. 281–293

Chapter 4
Engaging religious leaders to support HIV prevention and care for gays, bisexual men, and other men who have sex with men in coastal Kenya
Evans Gichuru, Bernadette Kombo, Noni Mumba, Salla Sariola, Eduard J. Sanders and Elise M. van der Elst
Critical Public Health, volume 28, issue 3 (June 2018) pp. 294–305

Chapter 5
Turning the gaze: challenges of involving biomedical researchers in community engagement with research in Patan, Nepal
Siân Aggett
Critical Public Health, volume 28, issue 3 (June 2018) pp. 306–317

Chapter 6

Chapter 7

Chapter 8

Chapter 9

Chapter 10

Chapter 11

For any permission-related enquiries please visit:
http://www.tandfonline.com/page/help/permissions

Contributors

Siân Aggett Global Studies, University of Sussex, Brighton, UK.

Crystal Biruk Department of Anthropology, Oberlin College, USA.

Virginia Bond School of Medicine, Ridgeway Campus, Zambart, Lusaka, Zambia; Department of Global Health and Development, London School of Hygiene & Tropical Medicine, Lusaka, Zambia.

Saheli Datta Department of Global Health and Social Medicine, King's College London, UK.

Evans Gichuru Kenya Medical Research Institute – Wellcome Trust Research Programme, Kilifi, Kenya.

Nils Graber Research Center Medicine, Sciences, Health, Mental Health, and Society (Cermes3), EHESS (Ecole des Hautes Etudes en Sciences Sociales), Paris, France.

Judith Green School of Population Health & Environmental Sciences, King's College London, UK.

Abhilasha Karkey Oxford University Clinical Research Unit, Kathmandu, Nepal.

Bernadette Kombo Kenya Medical Research Institute – Wellcome Trust Research Programme, Kilifi, Kenya.

Noni Mumba Kenya Medical Research Institute – Wellcome Trust Research Programme, Kilifi, Kenya.

Lieke Oldenhof and Rik Wehrens Institute of Health Policy and Management, Erasmus University, Rotterdam, The Netherlands.

Sharli Anne Paphitis Community Engagement Division, Rhodes University, Grahamstown, South Africa.

John Porter Departments of Clinical Research and Global Health and Development, London School of Hygiene & Tropical Medicine (LSHTM), UK.

Lindsey Reynolds Pivot Collective, Cape Town, South Africa; Stellenbosch University, Cape Town, South Africa.

Eduard J. Sanders Kenya Medical Research Institute – Wellcome Trust Research Programme, Kilifi, Kenya; Department of Global Health, Academic Medical Centre, University of Amsterdam, The Netherlands; Nuffield Department of Medicine, University of Oxford, UK.

Salla Sariola Sociology, University of Helsinki, Finland.

Andrew Scheibe TB HIV Care, Cape Town, South Africa; Department of Family Medicine, University of Pretoria, South Africa.

Shaun Shelly TB HIV Care, Cape Town, South Africa; Department of Family Medicine, University of Pretoria, South Africa.

Musonda Simwinga School of Medicine, Ridgeway Campus, Zambart, Lusaka, Zambia.

Gift Trapence Centre for the Development of People, Lilongwe, Malawi.

Elise M. van der Elst Kenya Medical Research Institute – Wellcome Trust Research Programme, Kilifi, Kenya; Department of Global Health, Academic Medical Centre, University of Amsterdam, The Netherlands.

Anna Versfeld WITS Institute for Social and Economic Research, University of the Witwatersrand, Johannesburg, South Africa; TB HIV Care, Cape Town, South Africa.

Janine Wildschut Mainline Drugs and Health, Amsterdam, The Netherlands; AIDS Foundation East West, Amsterdam, The Netherlands.

The ethics and politics of community engagement in global health research

Lindsey Reynolds and Salla Sariola

Introduction

Community engagement is an increasingly common component of scientific research, policy-making, ethical review, and technology design. Drawing on a growing consensus about the importance of community representation and participation for ethical research, a number of research institutions and funding bodies now promote, or even mandate, community engagement. Many researchers have also taken these normative expectations to heart, integrating diverse community engagement activities into their research practices. The increasing interest in and emphasis on community engagement can also be seen in the explosion of published articles over the last 30 years describing engagement activities across a wide variety of research areas. These include, to name only a small selection of a vast and growing literature: pandemic prevention and malaria control (e.g. Garrett, Vawter, Prehn, et al., 2009), genetics and genomics (e.g. Felt & Fochler, 2010), nanotechnology (e.g. Delgado, Kjølberg, & Wickson, 2010), patient advocacy (e.g. Rabeharisoa, Moreira, & Akrich, 2014), mental health (e.g. Campbell & Cornish, 2010), HIV prevention (e.g. Koen, Essack, Slack, et al., 2013), and biobanks (e.g. Papaioannou, 2011). It could be said that the ethos of community engagement and participation has become something of a zeitgeist in scientific research in recent decades.

Effective community engagement is increasingly understood by its proponents and practitioners to be essential for ensuring both instrumental objectives and moral ideals of scientific research. This is particularly the case when research is conducted across cultural, structural, or economic differences. Due to its historical origins and the nature of the research endeavour, global health research is often characterised by significant differences, and geographic distances, between researchers and those under study. Global health research projects and programmes are often initiated and led by researchers based in the Global North, where human capital and financial resources are concentrated, but rely heavily on the active participation of local researchers, practitioners, and participants in the Global South, where most 'global' health research and intervention is focused. The diversity of actors involved in large-scale transnational research collaborations and the broader 'background conditions' of global inequality and injustice that frame the field (King, Kolopack, Merritt, & Lavery, 2014) have led some researchers, funders, and policy-makers to conclude that community engagement is nothing less than a moral imperative (e.g. Nuffield Council on Bioethics, 2002; Emanuel, Wendler, Killen, & Grady, 2004).

It has been suggested that engagement has the potential to redress past harms; dissolve long-standing mistrust and suspicion; minimise the risk of further exploitation; compensate for or resolve existing differences in power, privilege, and positionality; allow for marginalised voices and experiences to be represented in the production of scientific knowledge; and ensure that research is relevant and impactful. To this end, its proponents suggest, engagement activities must aim to create meaningful partnerships between researchers and those who inhabit the social or physical spaces where research is being conducted (Israel, Schulz, Edith, & Becker, 1998). Through effective partnerships, proponents, and practitioners hope to move beyond interpersonal and structural inequalities and to foster genuine dialogue between researchers and study communities. Once partnerships are established, it is argued, ongoing dialogue and collaboration ensures that community members play an active role in shaping study design and implementation, thereby improving the quality of scientific research and ensuring its impact for marginalised communities and populations (MacQueen, Bhan, Frohlich, Holzer, & Sugarman, 2015).

Despite explicit objectives related to socially responsible knowledge production, inclusivity, and empowerment, practices of community engagement in global health research are not inherently democratising. As will be explored below, community engagement programmes can serve a wide variety of ends. Engagement activities can be used for purely instrumental goals – to gain community 'buy-in', to increase consent and study enrolment, or to ensure smooth research operations – rather than to achieve broader transformations in the politics and power dynamics of research. Further, despite the inclusive promises of community engagement, engagement practices can be exploitative or can serve to exclude already marginalised members of a community (Gbadegesin & Wendler, 2006). Instead of redressing ethical concerns around research, engagement activities can introduce new ethical and social challenges (Molyneux et al., 2016).

Rather than taking community engagement as a given, the papers in this edited collection highlight how processes of community engagement are shaped by particular local histories and social and political dynamics, and by the complex social relations between different actors involved in global public health research. By interrogating the everyday politics and practices of a wide variety of engagement activities across diverse contexts, the edited collection critically explores the social, political, and ethical dimensions of community engagement in global health research, policy-making, and practice. To this end, the contributors analyse the complex interactions between research organisations, governmental institutions, civil society actors, social movements, and interest groups that are involved in the conduct of community engagement. Further, by drawing out the conceptual underpinnings of community engagement and the contextual backgrounds that inform its conduct, contributions highlight how these relationships are shaped and reshaped by the particular economic, social, technological, bioethical, and developmental demands, pressures, and interests of biomedical research in diverse low-income settings. By including contributions from critical scholars as well as engagement practitioners, the edited collection draws together a set of papers that move between these spaces and approach the problem of 'engagement' from divergent perspectives, interrogating and expanding standard narratives of community engagement. Through this perspective, the collection also offers unique insights on broader issues of representation, power, and justice in global health.

Understanding the origins of community engagement

Despite the increasing emphasis on the importance of community engagement and participation in global health, relatively little attention has been paid to the origins of engagement and participation within global health. While community engagement in global health has had its own particular history and trajectory, many of its central ideologies, assumptions, motivations, and practices are linked to the broader histories and dynamics of what has sometimes referred to as the 'participatory turn' in scientific research. The 'participatory turn' has focused on interrogating and shifting the relationship between researchers and researched, 'expert' and 'non-expert', and between 'science' and 'society'[1] more broadly. While there is not sufficient space for an exhaustive review of the literature, we offer here a brief reading of the historical origins and underlying logics and assumptions of community engagement and participation across three interrelated fields: global and public health, international development, and science and technology studies (STS).

Promoting participation in health and development

As many historians of medicine have pointed out, the uneven distribution of power in the production of biomedical knowledge and the practice of biomedicine is not a new phenomenon, but has been a dominant feature of public health and medical research and intervention since the beginnings of modern biomedicine (e.g. Tilley, 2011). A concern with the involvement of local 'communities' and an emphasis on 'community-based' approaches to health promotion and service delivery first emerged in the 1960s as part of a broader commitment to strengthening primary health care systems health services in newly independent states (Cueto, 2004). The intent of the primary health care movement was to deliver locally appropriate health services that were universally accessible. This commitment was formalised in the language of 'community participation' in the 1978 Declaration of Alma-Ata (WHO, 1978).

Following a broader shift towards neoliberal paradigms in health and development in the 1980s, new global health collaborations began to replace state-focused, international health programmes (Brown, Cueto, & Fee, 2006). These new structures have also given rise to new governmental forms that have been instantiated through moral economies of responsibilisation and 'community ownership'. Despite increasing emphasis on community participation, recent social scientific literature has highlighted how historically rooted social dynamics and structural inequalities have continued to shape the conduct of health research in the Global South. Scholars have highlighted the social, political, ethical, and technical complexities of large-scale, transnational collaborations and explored the cross-regional relations that emerge between researchers, participants, and study communities in such spaces (e.g. Fairhead, Leach, & Small, 2006; Kelly, MacGregor, & Montgomery, 2017; Lavery et al., 2010; Molyneux & Geissler 2008; Montgomery & Pool, 2016; Montgomery, Sariola, Kingori, & Engel, 2017; Reynolds, Cousins, Newell, & Imrie, 2013; Tindana et al., 2015).

A somewhat similar process has unfolded in the field of international development, where community participation has increasingly become a central element of development programmes. Similar to the stated goals of community engagement in public health and medicine, participatory approaches in international development were intended to break the structural and social boundaries created by legacies of colonialism, racialised hierarchies, and inequalities and to allow for marginalised voices to be heard. The 1999 World Bank *Voices of the Poor* report, for example, explicitly aimed to place personal narratives of suffering at the heart of anti-poverty debates (Naraya, Patel, Schafft, Rademacher, & Koch-Schulte, 2000).

To involve communities in the conception and conduct of development interventions, development researchers and practitioners have deployed a variety of tools, perhaps most notably the methodology of Participatory Rural Appraisal (PRA) (Chambers, 1981). The approach has been widely used in international development programmes across Africa and Asia (e.g. Mukherjee, 1993). Moving beyond PRA, the model of community-based participatory research has aimed to involve communities more explicitly in the full process of knowledge production (Wallerstein, Duran, Oetzel, & Minkler, 2003). These approaches intend to bring the 'subjects' of development programmes into the process of defining the focus, procedures, and outcomes of interventions. Rather than simply being seen as subjects of research, local communities are understood to hold crucial social and technical knowledge that development practitioners should learn from to ensure that interventions are effective and responsive to community needs and interests (Mosavel, Simon, van Stade, et al., 2005). These approaches to participatory research have been taken up widely in global health research (e.g. Lorway, Thompson, Lazarus, et al., 2013).

A growing number of scholars, however, have critiqued the implementation of participatory approaches in development and global health, arguing that they fail to address underlying structural inequalities that shape relationships between diverse stakeholders in research endeavours (Cooke & Kothari, 2002). David Mosse has argued that participation can be a self-fulfilling strategy, in which those who are already successfully 'engaged' participate in the engagement process and modes of engagement are significantly constrained by existing power dynamics (Mosse, 2005). Cornwall (2010) and others have argued that by the mid-2000s, ideas of 'community' and 'participation' had become empty signifiers – deployed to signal a commitment to local perspectives, but often not carried through in any meaningful way.

Expert knowledge and trust in science

From the 1960s to the 1990s, a growing literature on 'public understanding of science' emphasised the importance of educating 'the public' about scientific developments. Bauer, Allum, and Miller (2007) have described how activities in this paradigm were often framed around 'a deficit model', which assumed that publics lack basic knowledge or understanding of science or scientific facts. The success of involving publics in this tradition was measured in terms of increases in scientific knowledge, or 'science literacy', amongst specific target groups (Wynne, 2006). Contemporary STS and public health scholars have questioned the underlying assumptions of this model regarding what forms of knowledge count as 'scientific' and how forms of knowledge are transfered.

Critical scholars have also raised concerns regarding the distribution of power in these top-down relations where 'science' is instantiated through the voices of 'experts', while 'society' is understood to be made up of 'non-expert' publics or communities (e.g. Davies, 2013; Gottweis, 2008; Stern & Green, 2008). Several authors have argued that such top-down approaches can cause harm, and pointed to the potentially transformative power of including lay publics in scientific knowledge production (Carlisle & Cropper, 2009; Ui, Heng, Yatsuya, et al., 2010). Critical scholars have brought attention to the everyday processes of knowledge production and power relations that play out in the design and conduct of science and the creation of policy (e.g. Hyysalo, Jensen, & Oudshoorn, 2016; Jasanoff, 2003; Leach, Scoones, & Wynne, 2005).

A few key moments of public crisis have reinforced the scholarly critique, shaken public trust in scientific knowledge and led to significant changes in science policies relevant to participation. In the UK, the mass burning of livestock due to foot and mouth disease in the 1990s resulted in a major 'crisis of trust' between government researchers, policy-makers, and 'lay' publics (UK House of Lords, 2000). Critical scholars argued that the crisis was caused by a failure of scientific institutions to take people's concerns and understandings seriously, treating them rather as passive recipients of knowledge (e.g. Jasanoff, 2003). To redress such concerns, they suggested, knowledge production and scientific policy-making must be democratised by involving publics in the design of research and policy, ensuring greater accountability, and redefining expertise and ownership. In 2000, in response to the crisis, the British House of Lords published a report entitled *Science and Society in 2000,* mandating community engagement and participation as an essential component of all research and science policy in the UK (UK House of Lords, 2000). Following on this advance a number of major research bodies (including the Royal Society and the Wellcome Trust) began to shift funding to community engagement activities. Similarly, public institutions in the UK began to encourage community participation in governance of research, design, and science policy.

In some contexts, social movements have managed to enact changes in priorities and practices of scientific research, representing an alternative, bottom-up model of 'science' and 'society' relations. The contest around scientific knowledge production and governmental funding in the early years of the HIV epidemic in the US is a notable example. In response to a relative lack of scientific and governmental attention to the 'gay men's health crisis' unfolding in the early 1980s, activist groups publicly demanded increases in funding and shifts in scientific priorities to better understand this new disease and develop treatments (Epstein, 1996). As innovative medical treatments were successfully developed and the HIV epidemic expanded worldwide, social movements began to focus on the question of access to anti-retroviral treatment. In South Africa, where the epidemic was causing a significant mortality and where no treatment was available, the Treatment Action Campaign carried out a successful campaign to demand access to ART in the public health care system (Heywood, 2009). In both contexts, in addition to demands for medical care, people living with HIV called on scientists and policy-makers to recognise the necessity of including their voices and perspectives in HIV research, policy, and programmes. More broadly, patient activist groups formed around a number of different health conditions have increasingly demanded a 'seat at the table' (Stern & Green, 2008) and an opportunity to be part of scientific knowledge processes and policy-making, embracing a motto of 'nothing about us without us'. In response to these demands and to broader ethical concerns, ethical guidelines have increasingly emphasised the importance of community engagement in global health and clinical trials research (e.g. Council for International Organizations of Medical Sciences (CIOMS), 2016; Nuffield Council on Bioethics, 2002).

The combination of ethical and policy mandates, increased levels of funding, recognition of the positive effects of engagement on the feasibility and quality of research, and continued demands from social movements and civil society actors for recognition and involvement have made community engagement an increasingly important component of global health research. At the same time, after nearly 40 years of scholarly research and implementation of community engagement and participation programmes in many contexts, some scholars have suggested that the field is undergoing a 'reflexive turn' (Chilvers, 2012). This turn is characterised by a growing awareness on the part of (some) engagement practitioners and researchers that, despite their lofty ideals, engagement activities have too often reproduced old models of top-down knowledge production and dissemination, privileged particular voices to the exclusion of others, and served to consolidate existing social inequalities. To take up these concerns and to seek new, transformative ways of engaging, the special issue brings together a diverse set of perspectives on the possibilities, promises, and pitfalls of community engagement in global health research.

Exploring the ethics and politics of community engagement

The edited volume emerges from a workshop which took place at the University of Oxford in September 2016. The aim of the workshop was to foster knowledge exchange between divergent actors working in and on community engagement, ranging from engagement practitioners and applied researchers to critical scholars. We focused in particular on facilitating knowledge translation from engagement practitioners and researchers based in the Global South. For many participants, their roles moved between practitioner, researcher, advocate, and activist. In addition to their different professional roles, workshop participants came from 21 countries and represented more than a dozen disciplinary backgrounds. Drawing together this diverse group of participants and authors fostered a rich, ongoing conversation that interrogated and moved beyond standard narratives of community engagement in global health.

To explore political, historical, and social tensions in the practice of engagement in global health research, the workshop, and the resulting papers have opened up a series of questions across multiple registers:

(1) First, engagement practitioners and critical research have addressed the descriptive realities of engagement: What counts as community engagement in global health research? Who are the players involved and what are their relationships like? Who is included and excluded from engagement activities? What makes engagement 'effective'? What are the challenges and tensions that emerge in everyday practices of engagement?

(2) Second, they have explored a set of broader normative questions: What constitutes ethical and just global health research, and how does engagement contribute to achieving this? What are the arguments for and against engagement? What exactly about engagement makes research more 'ethical'?

(3) Finally, authors have focused on the social and political contexts that shape (and are shaped by) engagement activities and global health research: How do engagement activities and global health research intersect with existing structures of power, local social relationships, and broader structural forces? What kinds of encounters and relationships are produced through these activities, and how do they (re)shape everyday social life? How do local historical specificities shape how the objectives of engagement are perceived and achieved?

The chapters included in this collection represent a selection of the papers circulated for the workshop itself, and are informed by the rich discussions that took place amongst participants.

Defining and refining the terms of engagement

The chapters in the edited collection demonstrate that the diverse (intended or unintended) effects of community engagement activities are determined in part by the various ways in which the concept of 'community engagement' itself is defined and enacted.

Firstly, the seemingly simple concept of 'community' is deployed in diverse ways in different social and political contexts, signalling intersecting ideas of power, belonging, and participation. The term has been widely used by researchers, development practitioners, anti-globalisation activists, and state and corporate actors, amongst others, to encode quite different understandings of and commitments to collective dynamics. The term is conceptualised very differently in diverse engagement programmes and everyday practices in global health. In some cases, communities are brought together simply as a result of physical proximity, by inhabiting a particular place, bounded by specific geographic, juridical, or bureaucratic borders. In other instances, communities are defined through a shared identity – such as sexual orientation or gender identity – that is of relevance to the engagement effort in some way. Alternatively, people involved in 'community engagement' activities may have had nothing in common except for a shared disease diagnosis or increased risk of contracting a specific disease. Or, in other instances, 'communities' may be constituted temporarily or fleetingly, as those who are brought together for a particular research activity or engagement event. These different understandings of the term can have important effects, particularly when definitions are imposed externally.

Similarly, the aims and practices of engagement are defined in multiple, differing, and sometimes overlapping ways. In many instances, engagement is conceived of as part of the ethical operations of a research institution and is thus conceptualised and practiced in order to satisfy the requirements of ethics board and others by ensuring 'community consent' or 'community representation' in research operations and decision-making. At other times, it is understood to be primarily a strategy for researchers and health practitioners to deliver scientific knowledge to communities through educational programmes and events. In other cases, engagement activities aim explicitly to shift or 'democratise' the process of knowledge production itself through bringing collectives together to shape research agendas, design and carry out research, and share their own insights. These forms of engagement can be linked more explicitly with activist agendas, aiming for structural transformations and social change. The various modes of 'engagement' also signal the diversity of individuals involved as engagement 'practitioners'.

Power and social relations

While several chapters offer 'case studies' from one country setting, most focus on transnational research programmes or projects that involve funders, researchers, or other stakeholders from different locations, thus embedding them within the 'global health research' establishment. In this complex space, the chapters in the collection highlight the importance of questions of power, positionality, authority, and privilege in the practice of community engagement.

Drawing on qualitative research with two community advisory boards (CABs) in Zambia, Simwinga, Porter, and Bond (2018) offer a critical exploration of the role of community advisory boards (CABs) in ensuring accountability between researchers and 'communities' in medical research. They describe how unequal power relations between researchers and CAB members and a lack of accountability on the part of researchers themselves produced powerful contradictions between stated goals and everyday operations of CABs (Simwinga et al., 2018). Relatedly, Aggett (2018) explores the quality and depth of involvement of researchers themselves in two participatory arts projects in Nepal. The author, an engagement practitioner herself, highlights how key contextual factors created 'logistical and attitudinal obstacles' to the genuine involvement of researchers in community engagement, including discomfort with creative methodologies, institutional and disciplinary hierarchies and priorities, and ambiguity from funders regarding the value of engagement.

Highlighting the complex dynamics of power and positionality in community engagement research in global health, the editorial by Karkey and Green (2018) responding to Aggett's article raises important questions about the limits, conflicting expectations, and politics of collaboration and the challenges of conducting critical ethnographies of community engagement. There is often a structuring assumption in critiques of global health research that researchers have power and communities do not, and that researchers from the global North have more power than those from the South. These critiques are often central to the rationale for engagement and participatory research in global health. However, who has the power to be seen as a legitimate producer of knowledge and to be heard is not always clear-cut when conducting research with powerful interlocutors. Clearly, effective engagement must involve not only lay populations but also researchers themselves, meaning that to critically study the processes of engagement is to study both 'up' and 'down.' Karkey and Green aptly describe the tensions involved in 'studying up' in the editorial, and raise critical questions about whose voice is prioritised through such processes. They also point out that processes of trust-building and community dialogue take time, and that critical researchers and engagement practition-ers who spend a fixed amount of time in local community contexts may miss some of this relational unfolding in the time scales of their own endeavours. To address such concerns, they argue for the po-tential value of collaborative and conversational forms of research and writing, which allow multiple positionalities and perspectives to be equally represented in academic publishing.

Interrogating the ends of engagement

The papers and broader conversations in the workshop and beyond highlight what might simplistically be seen as a set of arguments for and against community engagement. Some have focused on the positive attributes or potential of engagement work: as furthering normative ideals of democratisa-tion; shifting the ownership of science and redefining expertise; empowering individuals and addressing vulnerability; furthering normative ideals of democratisation; or promoting social justice. Van der Elst and colleagues (2018), for instance, describe a dialogue-based approach to addressing homophobic stigma amongst religious leaders in Kenya. In a context of extremely high rates of stigma towards sexual minorities, they argue, community engagement activities served not only to mobilise stakeholders around a public health research agenda, but also became sites for conflict resolution, trust building, sensitisation, and the sharing of different ontological and moral frameworks and perceptions (van der Elst et al., 2018). Implicit in their account is also a broader set of questions related to trust in scientific knowledge, colonial power relations, and competing moral and ethical frameworks.

Also working with a group of participants who often experience high rates of stigma and discrim-ination, Versfeld and colleagues (2018) reflect on the successes, limitations, and lessons learned from processes of community inclusion in a multi-city harm reduction service provision project for people who inject drugs in South Africa. They suggest that for many participants, active engagements through regular community advisory group meetings and 'consistent empathic responses' from the project team contributed to 'the (re)generation of a sense of a right to exist, comment on, and shape the world they live in' (Versfeld, Scheibe, Shelly, & Wildschut, 2018, p. 331). The authors point out at these impacts went well beyond the bounded, measurable aims of the public health intervention, speaking to the broader transformative potential of community engagement.

Others have offered more critical perspectives, exploring the ways that engagement work could be top-down and prescriptive; impose a form of governance or a political ideology; serve as 'window dress-ing' or a way of masking unequal power structures; potentially cause stigma, risk, or other unintended consequences; or produce or amplify experiences of inclusion and exclusion. Oldenhof and Wehrns (2018), for instance, describe how engagement activities for older people in a Dutch healthcare research programme produced new forms of exclusion for frail older people who lacked existing social, cultural, and symbolic capital. Further, despite their relative privilege, those who were included in engagement activities still expressed difficulties with effective participation in the evaluation and design of research. While focusing on a population who would generally be outside the gaze of 'global' health, the article offers important insights for global health research in its detailed analysis of everyday processes of inclusion and exclusion in community engagement work.

Competing arguments for and against community engagement, however, were not understood to be mutually exclusive. The papers and conversations highlighted how the same project could often move between different registers simultaneously. Despite concerns about the ways in which some engagement projects were rolled out, participants mostly agreed that engagement work was still essen-tial to ethical and just global health research. However, they suggested that assessing when and how engagement should be done ought to be weighed against broader, contextual needs, and objectives.

Community engagement and scientific knowledge production

Several chapters in the volume take up the tension between engagement as a set of practices intended to support and facilitate scientific research and engagement as an approach to transforming the production of scientific knowledge itself. The chapters offer quite different accounts of how communities might be engaged, or engage themselves, in the process of scientific research. The contribution by Biruk and Trapence (2018), written collaboratively by an American medical anthropologist and a Malawian researcher and activist working in an LGBTI rights organisation, argues for a broadening of the term 'research' itself to encompass activities often partitioned outside of the process of knowledge production through the use of language of 'engagement'. Once research comes to be understood in this more inclusive way, they suggest, it becomes possible to see other forms of risk and potential harm faced by LGBTI-identified volunteers working in this context. Through this perspective, the authors suggest, engagement must be understood

> not merely as strategy for improving ethics or enhancing research but as ambivalent process of building trust and suspicion and bringing benefits and harms to communities, many of which are invisible if we think only within normative bounded frames for engagement and ethics (Biruk & Trapence, 2018, p. 341).

Rather than focusing on scientists or practitioners engaging communities in the production or dissemination of research, Datta (2018) explores how 'communities' themselves engage with and interpret research. Datta describes how patients and their families share and evaluate disease-specific evidence related to experimental stem cell therapies on Facebook, in a sense removing scientists and clinicians from this process. Within these 'online communities', users combine scientific and experiential forms of evidence to produce more 'user-centred' form of science and 'user-to-user' engagement, motivated in part by an innate distrust in particular institutions and individuals involved in the production of scientific knowledge (Datta, 2018).

Drawing on ethnographic research in a series of oncology clinical trials in Cuba, Graber (2018) explores the meaning and practice of 'community engagement' in a political and social context where conventional notions of community engagement in global health research do not apply. Instead of a discrete set of activities designed to establish the legitimacy and efficiency of transnational research projects, the oncology trials implicitly engage communities and ensure that technological innovations are adapted to their needs by bringing cancer therapeutic innovations to primary health care (PHC) professionals, who already work in close relation to patients, relatives, and neighbourhoods (Graber, 2018). Community engagement in this context is thus embedded within the architecture and professional ethos of the PHC system itself. Graber encourages us to think beyond frameworks focused on discrete groups of 'stakeholders', and rather to see the diverse actors involved in global health research as embedded within shifting configurations of citizenship, medical practice, health research, and the nation state.

Reflecting on her own experiences of implementing a menstruation-related critical health project in South Africa, the commentary by Paphatis (2018) asks if engaged research practices can address underlying concerns with epistemic injustice in global health research. While highlighting some important successes of the engaged research process, she points out that many of her colleagues, the institution, and the project funders did not deem the more participatory forms of knowledge generation and dissemination as valid, valuable, or legitimate 'academically' (Paphatis, 2018). Instead, the project's more standard academic outputs, produced *without* active collaboration, remained the key metric of success. As a result, the project failed, in her assessment, to shift underlying power dynamics. To more effectively address epistemic injustice, Paphatis argues, requires researchers to challenge and transform their own ideas, practices, and power relations.

Next steps, lessons, and implications for policy and practice

The initial workshop on which this edited collection is based was conceived in response to a shared sense that the work of community engagement is too often an invisible form of labour in academic research – vital for its success, but taken for granted and not deemed as scientific (and thus, in many cases, not published). Relatedly, for many involved in the workshop and volume, the ability to participate in the conversation, to think critically about the practices of engagement, and to write up and eventually publish their work required ongoing negotiations around institutional politics, competing priorities, and the practical demands on their work. For some participants, practical and political challenges unfortunately meant they were eventually unable to complete or publish their papers.

Despite these challenges, this collection serves to highlight many of the key insights and themes of the broader collective process. The papers also push conversations around engagement and participation beyond their conventional framings to raise more radical questions about knowledge, power, expertise, authority, representation, inclusivity, and ethics. As several of our authors and participants highlighted, it is at times far too easy for radical, transformative politics to be depoliticised through their reification into structured sets of tools and interventions. The authors show that the belief in the emancipatory potential of participation doesn't always sit comfortably with the tools available to do community engagement and emphasise the need for more creative and inclusive modes of engagement.

Drawing on insights from the papers, broader conversations, and our own research in diverse sites of knowledge production in global health, we close by offering an initial set of recommendations for more transformative, inclusive, and meaningful community engagement in global health research:

(1)   Explore the messiness of engagement in the everyday and acknowledge the possibility for engagement to be both 'good' and 'bad'

As described above, assessments of the impact and importance of community engagement can fall into two categories – either engagement is seen to be empowering, democratising, and deconstructing or it is critiqued for being instrumental, tokenistic, and depoliticising. The authors in this collection have demonstrated, however, that the risks and benefits of community engagement are unpredictable, contextual, and relational: both ends of this dichotomy can co-exist within a single engagement project. This makes it difficult to standardise engagement and transfer the same models across geographic and social contexts.

This complexity does not mean, however, that those involved in engagement can release themselves from critical interrogation or self-reflexive duty. For engagement to be conducted effectively and ethically, it is vital to ask critical questions about the shifting everyday challenges of implementing engagement in diverse economic, social, political, and institutional contexts. By drawing attention to the importance of everyday experiences as a way of illuminating such problems, engaged and socially conscious research can illuminate the unequal structures of knowledge production and power that continue to dominate global health research. Such critical thinking can produce importance knowledge on the labour that goes into making global health research and engagement happen, and can suggest new, transformative modalities of community engagement in global health.

(2)   Ensure effective engagement across the knowledge production process

A key issue in the understanding and implementation of engagement in global health is that engagement is too often compartmentalised, or restricted to one part of the research process. Engagement rarely starts at the point of defining issues and shaping questions and extends through publication, dissemination, and policy-making. While we acknowledge that fully participatory research is not necessarily possible in all cases, implementing community engagement at only one moment of the knowledge production process is unlikely to achieve the kinds of emancipatory and transformative goals envisioned by its stronger proponents. The role of community engagement and participation must rather be thought throughout the knowledge production process. In particular, we would encourage research groups and collaborations, funders, and journals to consider how engaged, participatory research might carry through more effectively to academic publishing and authorship practices.

(3)   Develop and support training and skills building for community members and researchers

To work towards the transformative potential of community engagement and ensure that it causes no harm, it is necessary to develop the capacity of community members, practitioners, policy-makers, *and* academics to engage and participate in collective, transformative research partnerships. This training should entail not only the transfer of information about existing tools for engagement, but should also aim to encourage new and innovative approaches to knowledge production and implementation and to confront existing injustices and inequalities within the conduct of global health research. By enabling more effective community-led research, such programme could help to illuminate structural problems and provide spaces for young people and other vulnerable and excluded groups to contribute directly and meaningfully towards changing their community.

(4)   Promote transformative partnerships and collaborations

Much of the language around the importance of community engagement focuses on the values of building partnerships and collaborations. However, a key challenge to reframing North–South collaborations and promoting partnerships within the Global South remains the power imbalance created by the heavy reliance on Northern donors, who are thereby able to powerfully shape the terms of research projects and partnerships. Promoting partnerships without interrogating the terms of such arrangements can be counterproductive, creating new structures that (intentionally or unintentionally) exploit or disempower researchers and community partners in the Global South. Effective partnerships must explicitly acknowledge and aim to redress historically shaped structures of inequality in North–South collaborations. To do so will often require 'unequal' partnerships, where *more* opportunities and support are offered to some partners than others in order to redress existing inequalities. Further, partnerships should also entail a re-centring of research as a transformative social practice through embedding it in the local context, with leadership by and accountability to people living in the place the research is happening. These new modes of partnership and collaboration must privilege voices that have been historically underrepresented and undervalued and focus centrally on questions of epistemic and social justice.

(5)   Create incentive structures within research that encourage and reward genuine engagement

While an increasing number of funders encourage and fund engagement work and many research institutions have developed formal engagement programmes, there remain few incentives that encourage researchers to prioritise engagement and participatory research in their own professional lives. The current system of academic assessment and reward makes it challenging for many researchers to carry out the necessarily complex and time-consuming work of collaborative, participatory research and community engagement. Funding bodies and academic institutions should be aware of the (perhaps unintentional) roles they can play in discouraging engagement by rewarding particular forms of academic achievement (notably first/sole authorship of peer-reviewed journal articles), while undervaluing other kinds of contribution to knowledge production and dissemination. We would encourage institutional actors to re-evaluate and reframe their systems of assessment and reward to recognise the importance of participatory, collaborative research, and knowledge sharing.

Acknowledgement

We would like to acknowledge the generous input and involvement of Professor Mike Parker and other colleagues and members of the Global Health Bioethics Network, as well as Georgia Bladon from the Wellcome Trust.

Note

1.   We use this pairing as a shorthand, with full awareness that, as Franklin (1995) amongst others has argued, 'science' and 'society' are not distinct entities. For our purposes here, 'science' and 'society' are used as analytical concepts that allow us to examine particular processes of knowledge production and the diverse people and groups involved in.

Funding

The work was supported by the Wellcome Trust [grant number 201351/Z/16/Z]. Additional support was provided by the Global Health Bioethics Network, which is funded through a Wellcome Trust Strategic Award [grant number 096527].

References

Aggett, S. (2018). Turning the gaze: Challenges of involving biomedical researchers in community engagement with research in Patan, Nepal. *Critical Public Health, 28*(3), 306–317.

Bauer, M. W., Allum, N., & Miller, S. (2007). What can we learn from 25 years of PUS survey research? Liberating and expanding the agenda. *Public Understanding of Science, 16*(1), 79–95.

Biruk, C., & Trapence, G. (2018). Community engagement in an economy of harms: Reflections from an LGBTI-rights NGO in Malawi. *Critical Public Health, 28*(3), 340–351.

Brown, T. M., Cueto, M., & Fee, E. (2006). The World Health Organization and the transition from 'international' to 'global' Public Health. *American Journal of Public Health, 96*(1), 62–72. doi:10.2105/AJPH.2004.050831

Campbell, C., & Cornish, F. (2010). Towards a 'fourth generation' of approaches to HIV/AIDS management: Creating contexts for effective community mobilisation. *AIDS Care, 22*(sup2), 1569–1579.

Carlisle, S., & Cropper, S. (2009). Investing in lay researchers for community-based health action research: Implications for research, policy and practice. *Critical Public Health, 19*(1), 59–70.

Chambers, R. (1981). Rapid rural appraisal: Rationale and repertoire. *Public Administration and Development, 1*(2), 95–106.

Chilvers, J. (2012). Reflexive engagement? Actors, learning, and reflexivity in public dialogue on science and technology. *Science Communication, 35*(3), 283–310.

Cooke, B., & Kothari, U. (Eds.). (2002). *Participation, the new tyranny?* London: Zed Books.

Cornwall, A. (2010). Introduction. In A. Cornwall & D. Eade (Eds.), *Deconstructing development discourse: Buzzwords and fuzzwords.* Warwickshire: Oxfam Publishers.

Council for International Organizations of Medical Sciences (CIOMS). (2016). *International ethical guidelines for health-related research involving humans* (4th ed.). Geneva: Author

Cueto, M. (2004). The origins of primary health care and selective primary health care. *American Journal of Public Health, 94*(11), 1864–1874.

Datta, S. (2018). Emerging dynamics of evidence and trust in online user-to-user engagement: The case of 'unproven' stem cell therapies. *Critical Public Health, 28*(3), 352–362.

Davies, S. R. (2013). The rules of engagement: Power and interaction in dialogue events. *Public Understanding of Science, 22*(1), 65–79.

Delgado, A., Kjølberg, K. L., & Wickson, F. (2010). Public engagement coming of age: From theory to practice in STS encounters with nanotechnology. *Public Understanding of Science, 20*(6), 826–845.

Emanuel, E. J., Wendler, D., Killen, J., & Grady, C. (2004). What makes clinical research in developing countries ethical? The benchmarks of ethical research. *The Journal of Infectious Diseases, 189*(5), 930–937.

Epstein, S. (1996). *Impure science. AIDS, activism, and the politics of knowledge.* Berkeley, CA: University of California Press.

Fairhead, J., Leach, M., & Small, M. (2006). Where techno-science meets poverty: Medical research and the economy of blood in The Gambia, West Africa. *Social Science and Medicine, 63*, 1109–1120.

Felt, U., & Fochler, M. (2010). Machineries for making publics: Inscribing and de-scribing publics in public engagement. *Minerva, 48*(3), 219–238.

Franklin, S. (1995). Science as culture, cultures of science. *Annual Review of Anthropology, 24*(1), 163–184.

Garrett, J. E., Vawter, D. E., Prehn, A. W., DeBruin, D. A. & Gervais K. G. (2009). Listen! The value of public engagement in pandemic ethics. *The American Journal of Bioethics, 9*(11), 17–19.

Gbadegesin, S., & Wendler, D. (2006). Protecting communities in health research from exploitation. *Bioethics, 20*(5), 248–253.

Gottweis, H. (2008). Participation and the new governance of life. *BioSocieties, 3*(3), 265–286.

Graber, N. (2018). An alternative imaginary of community engagement: State, cancer biotechnology and the ethos of primary healthcare in Cuba. *Critical Public Health, 28*(3), 269–280.

Heywood, M. (2009). South Africa's treatment action campaign: Combining law and social mobilization to realize the right to health. *Journal of Human Rights Practice, 1*(1), 14–36.

Hyysalo, S., Jensen, T. E., & Oudshoorn, N. (Eds.). (2016). *The new production of users: Changing innovation collectives and involvement strategies.* London: Routledge.

Israel, B. A., Schulz, A. J., Edith, P. A., & Becker, A. B. (1998). Review of community-based research: Assessing partnership approaches to improve public health. *Annual Reviews of Public Health, 19*, 173–202.

Jasanoff, S. (2003). Technologies of humility: Citizen participation in governing science. *Minerva, 41*(3), 223–244.

Karkey, A., & Green, J. (2018). Speaking for others: Ethical and political dilemmas of research in global health. *Critical Public Health, 28*(5), 495–497.

Kelly, A. H., MacGregor, H., & Montgomery, C. M. (2017). The publics of public health in Africa. *Critical Public Health, 27*(1), 1–5.

King, K. F., Kolopack, P., Merritt, M. W., & Lavery, J. V. (2014). Community engagement and the human infrastructure of global health research. *BMC Medical Ethics, 15*(84), 1–6.

Koen, J., Essack, Z., Slack, C., Lindegger, G., & Newman P. A. (2013). 'It looks like you just want them when things get rough': Civil society perspectives on negative trial results and stakeholder engagement in HIV prevention trials. *Developing World Bioethics, 13*(3), 138–148.

Lavery, J. V., Tinadana, P. O., Scott, T. W., Harrington, L. C., Ramsey, J. M., Ytuarte-Nuñez, C., & James, A. A. (2010). Towards a framework for community engagement in global health research. *Trends in Parasitology, 26*(6), 279–283.

Leach, M., Scoones, I., & Wynne, B. (2005). *Science and citizens: Globalization and the challenge of engagement*. New York, NY: Zed Books.

Lorway, R., Thompson, L. H., Lazarus, L., du Plessis, E., Pasha, A., Mary, P. F., Khan, S., & Reza-Paul, S. (2013). Going beyond the clinic: Confronting stigma and discrimination among men who have sex with men in Mysore through community-based participatory research. *Critical Public Health, 24*(1), 73–87.

MacQueen, K., Bhan, A., Frohlich, J., Holzer, J., & Sugarman, J. (2015). Evaluating community engagement in global health research: The need for metrics. *BMC Medical Ethics, 16*(44), 1–9.

Molyneux, S., & Geissler, P. W. (2008). Ethics and the ethnography of medical research in Africa. *Social Science and Medicine, 67*(5), 685–890.

Molyneux, S., Sariola, S., Allman, D., Dijkstra, M., Gichuru, E., Graham, S., … Sanders, E. (2016). Public/community engagement in health research with men who have sex with men in sub-Saharan Africa: Challenges and opportunities. *Health Research Policy and Systems, 14*, 65.

Montgomery, C. M., & Pool, R. (2016). From 'trial community' to 'experimental publics': How clinical research shapes public participation. *Critical Public Health, 27*(1), 50–62.

Montgomery, C. M., Sariola, S., Kingori, P., & Engel, N. (2017). Global health and science and technology studies: Complacency and critique. *Science and Technology Studies, 30*(4), 1–13.

Mosavel, M., Simon, C., van Stade, D., & Buchbinder, M. (2005). Community-based participatory research (CBPR) in South Africa: Engaging multiple constituents to shape the research question. *Social Science & Medicine, 61*(12), 2577–2587.

Mosse, D. (2005). *Cultivating development: An ethnography of aid policy and practice*. London: Pluto.

Mukherjee, N. (1993). *Participatory rural appraisal: Methods and applications*. New Delhi: Concept Publishing Company.

Naraya, D., Patel, R., Schafft, K., Rademacher, A., & Koch-Schulte, S. (2000). *Voices of the poor: Can anyone hear us?* Washington DC: World Bank.

Nuffield Council on Bioethics (2002). *The ethics of research related to healthcare in developing countries*. Plymouth: Latimer Trend Group.

Oldenhof, L., & Wehrns, R. (2018). Who is 'in' and who is 'out'? *Participation of older persons in health research and the interplay between capital, habitus and field, Critical Public Health, 28*(3), 281–293.

Papaioannou, T. (2011). From consultation to deliberation? A qualitative case study of governing science and technology projects for the public good. *Critical Public Health, 22*(2), 235–251.

Paphatis, S. (2018). The possibility of addressing epistemic injustice through engaged research practice: Reflections on a menstruation related critical health education project in South Africa. *Critical Public Health, 28*(3), 363–372.

Rabeharisoa, V., Moreira, T., & Akrich, M. (2014). Evidence-based activism: Patients', users' and activists' groups in knowledge society. *BioSocieties, 9*(2), 111–128.

Reynolds, L., Cousins, T., Newell, M.-L., & Imrie, J. (2013). The social dynamics of consent and refusal in HIV surveillance in rural South Africa. *Social Science & Medicine, 77*, 8e125.

Simwinga, M., Porter, J., & Bond, V. (2018). Who is answerable to whom? Exploring the complex relationship between researchers, community and Community Advisory Board (CAB) members in two research studies in Zambia. *Critical Public Health, 28*(3), 318–328.

Stern, R., & Green, J. (2008). A seat at the table? *A study of community participation in two Healthy Cities Projects, Critical Public Health, 18*(3), 391–403.

Tilley, H. (2011). *Africa as a living laboratory. Empire, development, and the problem of scientific knowledge, 1870–1950*. Chicago, IL: University of Chicago Press.

Tindana, P., de Vries, J., Campbell, M., Littler, K., Seeley, J., Marshall, P., … Parker, M. (2015). Community engagement strategies for genomic studies in Africa: A review of the literature. *BMC Medical Ethics, 16*(24), 1–12.

Ui, S., Heng, L., Yatsuya, H., Kawaguichi, L., Akashi, H., & Aoyana, A. (2010). Strengthening community participation at health centers in rural Cambodia: Role of local non-governmental organizations (NGOs). *Critical Public Health, 20*(1), 97–115.

UK House of Lords. (2000, March) *Select committee on science and technology: Science and society*. London: House of Lords.

van der Elst, E., Gichuru, E., Kombo, B., Mumba, N., Sariola, S., & Sanders, E. (2018). Engaging religious leaders to support HIV prevention and care for gay and bisexual men, and other men who have sex with men in Coastal Kenya. *Critical Public Health, 28*(3), 294–305.

Versfeld, A., Scheibe, A., Shelly, S., & Wildschut, J. (2018). Empathic response and no need for perfection: Reflections on harm reduction engagement in South Africa. *Critical Public Health, 28*(3), 329–339.

Wallerstein, N., Duran, B., Oetzel, J., & Minkler, M. (Eds.). (2003). *Critical issues in developing and following CBPR principles*. San Fransisco, CA: Jossey Bass.

WHO. (1978). *Primary health care: Report of the international conference on primary health care, Alma-Ata USSR 6–12 September 1978*, Geneva.

Wynne, B. (2006). Public engagement as a means of restoring public trust in science – hitting the notes, but missing the music? *Public Health Genomics, 9*(3), 211–220.

An alternative imaginary of community engagement: state, cancer biotechnology and the ethos of primary healthcare in Cuba

Nils Graber

ABSTRACT

This paper analyzes a form of community engagement that differs from the way it is usually conceived and practiced in the domain of global health. This story takes place in the Cuban context and more specifically in a recent programme of oncology clinical trials implemented in primary healthcare (PHC) centres. By considering both the genealogy of this program and local interactions between PHC professionals and patients and their close relatives, I show that, in the context of Cuban socialist biomedicine, community engagement emerges as an implicit practice that forms part of the PHC professional ethos. I explore the ways cancer biomedicine is adapted in order to address specific needs and demands related to public acceptance of cancer in the Cuban society, diagnostic communication and palliative care. I argue that the way community engagement is enacted within Cuban socialist biomedicine is alternative to the global health dominant paradigm since it does strengthen existing relations between citizenry, health professions and public health infrastructures. Finally, by questioning the specificity of such socialist approach to community engagement, I suggest it greatly contributes to global health literature, because it creates continuity within existing state infrastructures rather than bypasses them, and, furthermore, offers a unique vantage on the treatment of chronic disease.

Introduction

In 2009, one of the main Cuban biotechnology centres – the Center of Molecular Immunology (CIM[1]) – partnered with the Ministry of Public Health (Minsap) to launch a clinical trials pilot-programme. This programme was designed to test locally developed cancer immunotherapies – i.e. treatments that act upon the immune system to destroy tumour cells – in primary healthcare (PHC) centres called 'polyclinics'. The programme consisted of what local researchers term 'pragmatic' clinical trials designed to assess not only the effectiveness of the treatments but also whether cancer care could be integrated into the polyclinics, while oncology had previously been exclusively practiced in hospitals. The trials aimed to develop a strategy for implementing cancer immunotherapies in about one polyclinic per municipality (about 124 institutions) on the island. They would permit thousands of patients to access these cutting-edge drugs close to home. Furthermore, PHC practitioners, namely family doctors and nurses, who are trained to adapt their practices to people's needs by living in community settings, would administer the treatment (Brotherton, 2012; Feinsilver, 1993).

I attempt to shed light on the form of 'community engagement' taking place through these PHC oncology trials in Cuba. I suggest that these engagements differ from the ways the term is usually conceived and practiced in global health research. There, community engagement usually takes place in the context of transnational research projects and humanitarian interventions marked by long histories of colonialism and exploitation (King, Kolopack, Merritt, & Lavery, 2014). In order to establish the legitimacy and efficiency of research projects, community engagement is intended to foster 'dialogue' with targeted communities, which is then (theoretically) fed back into the project design and implementation (MacQueen, Bhan, Frohlich, Holzer, & Sugarman, 2015). Although bioethical literature on community engagement attempts to avoid a reification of the notion of 'community' by considering a plurality of 'stakeholders' with different interests and values (King et al., 2014; Lavery et al., 2010), a feature of community engagement that is often overlooked is the way in which it often brackets off 'the community' from state institutions (Pfeiffer, 2003). This draws on a more general conceptualization of global health as a field of research and interventions that emerged in the late 1990s by replacing the old regime of 'international heath' (Brown, Cueto, & Fee, 2006), and is now characterized by the dominant role of the World Bank, international NGOs, university lead programs, philanthropic organizations, and private firms (Birn, 2014; Lakoff, 2010). Even if global health interventions attempt to be responsive to communities' needs and foster 'civil society' participation, ethnography-based scholarship has shown that such interventions usually take place within short-term programmes, where coordination with local health professionals and institutions is weak, producing a fragmented healthcare systems in many Southern countries (Crane, 2013; Pfeiffer, 2003). Furthermore, global health interventions tend to focus on 'technology delivery' with a poor understanding of people's social life, temporalities and 'local knowledge' (Adams, Burke, & Whitmarsh, 2014; Biehl & Petryna, 2013) As part of a neoliberal agenda ushered in by 'structural adjustment' in the 1980s, global health interventions have favoured market-based reforms over state-run public programs (Pfeiffer & Chapman, 2010; Prince & Marsland, 2014).

I explore the distinctive form of community engagement at stake in contemporary Cuban biomedicine and its linkage with state socialism. Socialist and post-socialist health contexts have been widely overshadowed within global health literature. Perhaps this can be explained by Cold War representations that reified a binary opposition between 'socialist' and 'capitalist' societies (Geltzer, 2012; Vargha, 2014). Indeed, scholars have shown how in post-soviet countries global health programs were explicitly attempting to eradicate socialist state legacies envisioned as essentially authoritarian and repressive (Keshavjee, 2014), sometimes associated with 'community participation' models to 'export democracy' (Atlani-Duault, 2008; Koch, 2013). To that extent, Cuba, its so-called 'medical internationalism,' its local biotechnology industry giving priority to address national needs (Reid-Henry, 2010), and its commitment to a universal healthcare system based on PHC has a unique place within health globalization (Burke, 2013; Graber, 2013). In a Cuban context, communities are defined at the level of neighbourhood (*barrio*), which is not only an administrative unit, but a central place of social life where people share a common experience of the health system (Brotherton, 2012; Gibbon, 2013). Each neighbourhood includes a health office (*consultorio*) where a family doctor and nurse work, and frequently live. They are usually perceived as part of the community by local people (*Ibid.*). While existing scholarship has shown how communities are deeply entangled within state health infrastructures, the way they are engaged remains unclear.

Following Kelly (2011), I consider the PHC cancer immunotherapy clinical trials as a 'public experiment' that transforms PHC infrastructures through the process of inserting and assessing oncology innovation. I will show how community engagement is enacted by PHC professionals in their attempt to constantly adapt cancer biomedicine to the communities' needs. I argue that this form of community engagement represents an alternative imaginary to the one fostered in the global health context because it is building upon existing configurations of care, medical citizenship, health professions, and state infrastructures. By focusing on the ways PHC professionals adapt cancer biomedicine to local people's needs, in a context of scarce resources, I follow Livingston's (2012, p. 96) argument about the professional ethos of care that does not only reflect an ethical dimension, but also a political one that prolongs the 'commitment of the state to care for its people.' This article is organized in two parts. First, by outlining the genealogy of the PHC oncology clinical trials, I show how this programme, which is enmeshed within the PHC professional ethos, implicitly integrates community engagement. Secondly, I present ethnographical material that sheds light on the ways family doctors and nurses set the conditions for the emergence of new individual and collective cancer experiences, in a context marked by both pervasive paternalism and cancer stigma (Gibbon, 2011, 2013). Moreover, I emphasize the PHC professionals' engagement with community to provide continuity between curative and palliative care. To conclude, I discuss the differences and overlap between the form of community engagement I have explored in the context of Cuban socialist biomedicine and the global health paradigm.

Methodology

This paper draws on research (between 2014 and 2016) conducted on the trajectory of cancer immunotherapy in Cuba. It is an ethnography of PHC clinical trial implementation. Hosted by the Cuban National Institute of Oncology (INOR), my research contributes to local efforts to understand the impact of this 'process,' by considering social aspects of institutional change, professional relations, and the experiences of PHC practitioners, patients and their families. I collaborated with the Health and Technology Assessment (HTA) team at the Centre of Molecular Immunology (CIM) that implemented social epidemiology approaches focusing mostly on assessing efficacy and ensuring product delivery. I conducted 58 interviews (33 recorded) related to the PHC clinical trials: 7 with oncologists, 8 with CIM researchers, 3 with public health and regulatory authorities, 22 with PHC practitioners (7 doctors, 7 nurses, 4 psychologists and 4 laboratory technicians) and 16 with patients (8 included at hospitals, 8 at the polyclinics). The PHC sites were selected according to direct relations I established with PHC practitioners during meetings and workshops about the trials. I was also able to undertake observations of consultations at both polyclinics and hospitals. Ethical clearance was obtained at both my host (INOR) and home institution (XXX). In an attempt to grasp territorial differentiation, about half of the data were collected in Havana and the remaining in the provinces of Villa Clara and Santiago de Cuba. The material was analyzed according to a biosocial medical anthropology perspective in order to understand how local practices within an on-going process are providing new accounts of wider politico-economical configurations of global health (Janes & Corbett, 2009).

The PHC oncology clinical trials: professional ethos and institutional framework

Community engagement in Cuba: from mass-mobilization to a community healthcare ethos

Since the Cuban revolution in 1959, community engagement has been a core component in the building of a national health system guided by socialist development vision that was grounded on the principles of health as a human right (WHO, 1975). Yet, community engagement has taken different forms. In the first two decades of the revolutionary era, health development politics were inspired by the Soviet health system and relied mainly on a mass-mobilization model (Feinsilver, 1993). First, the national health system was built through the training of a huge numbers of health professionals that were sent to rural areas to build basic medical infrastructures – often from scratch. Second, the whole Cuban population was mobilized through newly established revolutionary 'mass organizations'[2] to build health infrastructures and implement prevention campaigns like vaccination (Beldarraín, 2013; WHO, 1975). Under the mass-mobilization model collective efforts were limited to the efficient delivery of healthcare services on the island and were frequently expressed by military metaphors like 'the battle against dengue' or the creation of an 'army of white coats' (Feinsilver, 1993).

Community engagement took on another dimension in the 1980s with the creation of the 'family doctors and nurses' program' (*Médico y Enfermera de la Familia*, MEF). The MEF programme initiated the creation of *consultorios* or neighbourhood health offices, responsible for the health of an 'area' of about 120 households. This model relies on the *sectorialization* of the national health system: each consultorio is linked to a polyclinic, which is further linked to a hospital[3]. However, in the MEF model, 'community' does not only refer to a target population of healthcare delivery. Rather it is defined above all as a singular group of people sharing a common experience in a territorial unit (Brotherton, 2012). Following the Alma-Ata Declaration's principles, the MEF programme builds on a holistic conception of health and a participatory approach to adapt healthcare to local communities' needs (Feinsilver, 1993; Reed, 2008). Formal participation was promoted by the inclusion of 'community representatives' within PHC advisory boards that organized health services planning and implementation. Board representatives were usually elected members of the 'Neighbourhood Popular Councils', instances created in 1976 as the local basis of political power (Feinsilver, 1993, p. 81).

Besides a formal participatory framework, the MEF program permitted the stabilization of the *PHC professional ethos*. Considered as a practical feature rather than an explicit set of rules, the professional ethos is acquired through training and everyday practice (Fassin, 2008). By initiating the specialty of 'Integral General Medicine' (MGI) as a mandatory diploma in medical training, which includes a residency at a consultorio, the MEF program made the doctor community–patient relationship a central feature of PHC (Brotherton, 2012). In daily practice, family doctors and nurses conduct at-home visits to carry out epidemiological surveillance and attend to the social environment of sick persons (by considering the family context, housing situation and socio-economic situation among others dimensions) (Batista Moliner & González Ochoa, 2000). As anthropologists pointed out (see Andaya, 2009; Brotherton, 2012; Gibbon,2011, 2013), family doctors are frequently granted a status of local leader due to their prestige and knowledge of neighbourhood life. Thus, perceived as role model, they foster informal forms of participation to voice communities' concerns about medical and non-medical problems (such as housing, street cleanliness, delinquency, etc.). Another aspect of the PHC ethos is multidisciplinary practice: each community is followed by a 'basic work group' (*grupo basico de trabajo*) composed notably of a general practitioner, a nurse, a gynaecologist, a psychologist, a statistician and a social worker.

In the Post-Soviet era, marked by the 'Special Period' crisis of the 1990s (when the economy collapsed and the US reinforced its embargo), the whole public health system was threatened. Until today, there have been pervasive shortages and a surge of social inequalities that have affected the state's ability to meet local needs and demands considerably. Nevertheless, the public health infrastructures and PHC ethos have remained, which may explain why the main health indicators did not deteriorate (Spiegel & Yassi, 2004). Furthermore, my ethnography, which coincides with precedent anthropological work, indicates that the Cuban population still perceives family doctors and nurses as part of their community. As scholars suggest (Andaya, 2009; Brotherton, 2012), in the Post-Soviet context, the fact that relationships between doctors and communities were increasingly marked by an economy of 'favours and gifting', has perpetuated the PHC ecology rather than undermined it.

In the current context, formal community engagement frameworks, such as the mass mobilization one or the more participatory one linked to the Alma-Ata Declaration, are still at play in the Cuban health system. Yet, they are mainly taking place in infectious disease management, especially in the 'fight' against mosquito-borne diseases (Brotherton, 2012, pp. 125–127; Sanchez et al., 2009). However, in the case of chronic disease management, particularly cancer, I suggest that community engagement in Cuba finds its most powerful expression as an implicit practice forming part of the PHC professional ethos that is enacted in the direct relations between PHC practitioners, patients and their families.

'Bringing cancer biotechnology to the street corner': an implicit form of community engagement

Launched in 2009, the PHC oncology clinical trials sprang from a new Comprehensive National Cancer Control Program (PICC) implemented in 2004 to strengthen, among other things, the integration of the national biopharmaceutical industry with the whole health system, including at the PHC level (Romero, 2009). This strategy addresses problems of access to cancer care in a context dramatically marked by transport difficulties and a lack of imported technology inherited from the Special Period crisis. While the PHC level had already been involved in cancer prevention and screening, the PICC's novelty is treatments within polyclinics.

The PHC oncology clinical trials programme was designed by the CIM in coordination with Minsap as an innovative public health experiment attempting to transform advanced cancer into chronic disease manageable at the level of PHC (Lage & Crombet, 2011). It is grounded in cancer immunotherapies, a field the Cuban biotechnology industry has investigated since the 1980s (Lage, 2008; Reid-Henry, 2010). Currently, CIM produces both 'therapeutic vaccines' – generating cancer antigen-specific immune reactions – and monoclonal antibodies targeting tumour biomarkers. Until today, three PHC cancer protocols have been carried out; all test locally developed biopharmaceuticals for advanced (metastatic) non-small cells lung cancer (NSCLC). This choice was mainly informed by public health objectives, because lung cancers account for about 20% of the overall mortality by cancer in Cuba (Minsap, 2014). Considering the lack of accessible treatments for NSCLC, especially in developing countries, this focus is also informed by CIM's exportation strategy. This programme highlights the 'socialist' dimension of the Cuban biotechnology industry, which relies on the articulation between market-driven exporting strategies and public health programmes at the national level and through South–South agreements (Reid-Henry, 2010). Regarding the PHC oncology clinical trials, a CIM's executive expresses its political mandate in the following terms:

> A [private] firm is not interested in evaluating the effect of its drug in an open-population. Furthermore, I have always said that the difference between CIM and a pharmaceutical firm is that…stock exchange restricts to approve a drug and then sell it, it does not care about *coverage* and or *social benefit* [my emphasis] neither do they care about reducing mortality. No. Our goal is really that in Cuba people will die less from lung cancer, knowing it is the first cause of death … (…) We need to reach to make compatible chronic treatment with quality of life and considering the insertion of the patient in its work, social, and familiar life. Then it's why we need to bring it to the street corner with a very safe drug …

The CIM executive emphasizes the industry engagements necessary to conduct phase IV clinical trials, which are post-approval protocols designed to assess the impact of a drug in the 'real-life' settings as opposed to the standardized procedure of classical randomized clinical trials (RCT). For trials in an 'open-population', there is no predefined sample's size limit and inclusion criteria are expanded to include elderly patients suffering from co-morbidities who are usually excluded from RCT. Such trials are rarely conducted by private firms, since they usually do not provide economic value (Davis & Abraham, 2011), but are used in global health programs (Montgomery, 2017). In the interview, the executive expresses CIM's political mandate through a commitment to ensure 'population coverage' and to 'bring' the product within patients' social environments. Furthermore, the excerpt emphasizes the importance of developing drugs that are very safe and can be delivered in the health system, including PHC. This shows how the industry is concerned with the products' quality and delivery. The team of social epidemiologists at CIM, with which I collaborated as a social scientist, is dedicated to evaluate the drugs' impact in terms of effectiveness and coverage. These researchers, who conceived the protocols in collaboration with oncologists and Minsap's experts, do not promote community engagement as an explicit feature. Rather, community engagement is envisioned as an implicit practice enacted by 'bringing' therapeutic innovations to PHC professionals.

A professional demand to 'treat cancer patients in the community'

A key component of the new PICC, one that was pivotal for building capacity for the PHC oncology clinical trials, was the creation of a Certificate of oncology for PHC professionals (*Diplomado Básico Nacional de Control del Cáncer*). The certificate began as a pilot program in 2007 in Havana and centred on prevention, screening and palliative care. From 2009 it expanded to include clinical trials and basic oncology. Health authorities sent a call for application in every polyclinic selected for the trials to establish a 'PHC research team' composed of a family doctor, a nurse, a psychologist, a pharmacist and a laboratory technician. Hundreds of PHC professionals applied to the certificate program, which highlighted the demand for learning more about cancer care. Thus, a family doctor involved in the trial explained:

In the medical training there is nothing, no specific program on the cancer theme. Then, really every doctor, when you graduate, when you are in the *consultorio*, you begin to see patients who really have cancer. They are in their household, at home. This is why it was a demand of knowledge as such from family doctors, to know something related to cancer in order to treat these patients that you have in the community.

This excerpt emphasizes the demand by PHC practitioners for specific knowledge and tools to care for cancer patients whom they follow at *consultorio* and polyclinics. The doctor points to the paucity of cancer care training in the general medical education. Until very recently while the general practitioner specialty (MGI) emphasized community healthcare it did not prepare practitioners to manage cancer patients. Cancer was exclusively envisioned as a set of diseases requiring complex technology and invasive treatments circumscribed to the spaces of specialized services at hospitals or research institutes. PHC practitioners frequently expressed a prevailing 'fear' of cancer patients, which points to the wider 'cultural stigma of cancer' in Cuban society that Gibbon explores (2013, p. 13) in her ethnography about community genetics of breast cancer on the island. In my hospital ethnography, I also found a strong 'paternalism' in Cuban oncology: patients are often not informed when diagnostics reveal malignancy. Oncologists frequently justified this non-communication of the diagnosis (or at least euphemization) with reference to the common belief among patients that 'cancer equals death'. Informing patients about a serious condition could lead to a trauma, depression or even suicide. At the same time, however, oncologists systematically inform patients' family members about the diagnosis (and usually prognosis). As it has been showed elsewhere in the Global South (Sariola & Simpson, 2011), 'medical paternalism' and 'family-centredness' reveal other conceptions of the human subject often at odds with Western biomedicine's 'autonomous agent.'

In Cuban socialist biomedicine, paternalism could seem a normal and desired feature, as the state emphasizes its responsibility to preserve and better the health of its citizens. My ethnography in polyclinics sheds light on a more complex picture: the PHC professionals are enacting community engagement with the intent build new individual and collective experiences of cancer that transcends cancer stigma and challenges paternalism.

Local practices of community engagement: integrating cancer chronic treatment within the PHC

The vaccine form: normalizing the figure of the cancer patient through technology adaptation

In the main corridor of a polyclinic in Old Havana, I am waiting for Dr María,[4] the family doctor in charge of a cancer clinical trial who offered me the opportunity to be present at her consultation. She proposed that I sit next to the vaccination room (*vacunatorio*), the place where she will attend the patient, who is a bit late today. I am surrounded by young children accompanied by their mothers, waiting to be vaccinated against infectious diseases. The nurse at the *vacunatorio* calls them one at a time, which generally provokes the shouts of the toddlers. Suddenly, Dr María comes back, accompanied by an old lady, who is having trouble walking. She is giving one arm to the doctor, the other to a man, probably her son. They slowly enter the *vacunatorio* and Maria invites me to follow them. I begin to talk with the patient and her son while the nurse is preparing the intravenous infusion of the monoclonal antibody Nimotuzumab. While she is being injected with what is termed a 'serum' (*suero*), Josefina, the old lady, explained to me how her life was shattered when she was diagnosed with 'such a disease' two years ago at a hospital. The interview is interspersed by the children shouting as the nurse continues to vaccinate next to us. (*Fieldnotes, Havana,* January 2016)

At first glance, this observation seems to show that cancer immunotherapy is administered in a way that echoes the prophylactic vaccination model – long-standing PHC interventions familiar to the Cuban population.[5] The treatment is administered in the *vacunatorio*; the nurse who administers the cancer biological to the elderly woman is also the one who vaccinates children. The substance administered was not really a cancer 'therapeutic vaccine' (see Lage, 2008), which is injected intramuscularly like a prophylactic vaccine, but an intravenous infused monoclonal antibody. Yet, its effect was also referred to as an 'immunization'. In spite of these several analogies, the way cancer immunotherapy is administered to Josefina substantially differs from the way the young children surrounding her are immunized. While the toddlers are the passive targets of a mass vaccination campaign, the woman is an active actor of her treatment who can negotiate its meaning and its modes of administration.

Josefina is aware that the vaccine is a *therapeutic* one, which is treating but not preventing cancer. As we initially talked in an elusive way about her 'disease', she explained to me that she never smoked but that her husband did, and added: 'I am part of the passive smokers who get lung cancer.' Using the term 'cancer' in this consultation, next to young mothers and children, she is making the disease and her illness publicly visible and meaningful, which overtakes the cultural stigma of cancer as a disease equating death. The vaccine form, which makes the treatment familiar and understandable by echoing prophylactic vaccination, contributes to instilling a new representation of cancer as a disease that can be 'controlled' through repeated 'immunizations'; Dr Maria proudly indicated to me that Josefina is getting her 'number 12', which means she has been included in the protocol now for about 24 weeks.

This excerpt also shows how acts of 'tinkering' (Mol, Moser, & Pols, 2010) are used to integrate cancer immunotherapy within the socio-spatial dynamics of polyclinics, which facilities the normalization of the figure of the (lung) cancer patient within the community (including young mothers and their children). In such settings, patients' demands are more likely to be met than in the highly structured space of a hospital's oncology service. Thus, as Dr María explained to me later, she usually tries to conduct oncological consultations at another room in the basement of the polyclinic, behind closed doors, in order to get more privacy. But given that Josefina prefers the *vacunatorio*, because it is more easily accessible and of its public dimension, Dr Maria was willing to respect her wish.

Therapeutic vaccination, then, is not implemented as part of a vertical program designed to target a specific disease, as is common in mass-vaccination campaigns (Wailoo, Livingston, Epstein, & Aronowitz, 2010), but as a negotiated intervention, shaped by both past interactions between PHC professionals, cancer patients and the wider community of people at the polyclinic. As an implicit practice embedded within care interactions, community engagement is going beyond the national industry's political mandate to delivering efficient and safe drugs. Dr Maria is adapting biomedicine to make cancer an understandable and accepted disease within the community that is bound to her polyclinic.

Dr Flora's huequito: fostering the emergence of a community experience of cancer

At a polyclinic situated in a working-class suburb in Eastern Havana, I met Dr Flora and two of her patients included in the PHC clinical trial. Dr Flora has been a family doctor here for more than twenty years and still works at a *consultorio* located in the same neighbourhood where she lives. She and her patients call the place where the clinical trial take place their 'small corner' (*el huequito nuestro*). Because there was no consultation room available in the polyclinic, Dr Flora managed to set up a specific consultation in two small abandoned administrative offices in the polyclinic's backyard. She moved some old benches onto the patio to make a waiting room. One office is designed for vaccinations and the storage of medical records and protocols. The other is not only set up as an oncology consultation room (where walls are covered by cancer prevention messages and posters), but as a more intimate place with Flora' souvenirs and family photos on the shelves, and a Cuban coffee maker. Dr Flora's *huequito* highlights local initiatives by PHC professionals designed to re-arrange often-scarce clinical resources and spaces to produce a community experience of cancer. It is a semi-open place, suited to patients and their relatives, but also to other people from the neighbourhood who are worried about having a cancer (Flora usually receives them before the clinical trial's consultation).

The following excerpt of fieldwork's notes sheds light on how the cancer patients' voices are expressed and promoted at the *huequito*:

> Jorge, a former technician, is 58 years old and has received the therapeutic vaccine Cimavax-EGF for 6 years. He is one of the oldest survivors of the clinical trials. Rogelio, a thin old man who still works as a carpenter, has been included for two years in another protocol (a phase III non-inferiority trial), in which he has been randomly allocated to the arm receiving a monoclonal antibody.

The two patients are talking together with me about the conflicting situations with their family regarding diagnostic communication and therapeutic decisions. Rogelio really learnt that he had lung cancer when he was asked to participate in the clinical trial by his oncologist. His family did not want to include him, thinking that the chemotherapy and radiotherapy cycles he had previously received were enough. He decided to include himself despite his family's reticence. He signed the consent form protocol and asked a neighbour to sign it (as it is required to get a witness signature). After having started the treatment at the polyclinics, Dr Flora asked to meet his family members in order to explain to them the aims and process of this clinical trial. But even if they understand better, they still do not accompany Rogelio to the consultations.

Rogelio said to Jorge: 'They could not, they had to accept what I said. This is normal. This is me struggling for life. You cannot let me die!' Jorge answered him in a more nuanced way about patient autonomy. He says: 'In some cases it can be negative, in others positive. It depends on the person's conscience. Do you understand? It depends of how you are prepared, of your psychology, your constitution'. Jorge explains that he was himself 'not prepared to know' he had cancer when he was at the hospital receiving chemotherapy. He could really accept the diagnostic when he came to Flora's consultation. (*Fieldnotes, Havana's Eastern suburb, May 2016*)

Flora's *huequito* showcases how a form of community cancer care is established through PHC practitioners' local initiatives to arrange new social clinical spaces. The conversation between Rogelio and Jorge draws attention to the different perceptions of notions such as 'autonomy' or 'collective ethics' among Cuban patients. In Rogelio's case, the informed consent, as a device centred on autonomy principles as opposed to 'family-centeredness' ethics (Sariola and Simpson, 2011), represented an opportunity for self-affirmation against his family's will. Conversely, Jorge considers it unethical to reveal the cancer diagnosis to a sick person who is not 'psychologically' prepared. In his case, informed consent was not of any help; he could only accept the disease through a spiritual practice (meditation) but also through the interactions at Flora's *huequito*, with both his her family doctor and other patients.

Despite their contrasting views on medical paternalism, Jorge and Rogelio value Dr Flora as a mediating figure. In both cases, Dr Flora plays a crucial role by engaging intra-familial tensions and personal trauma caused by cancer diagnosis and treatments. By exploring each situation's medical and social components, she helps patients become actors beyond the formal informed consent. It is important to stress that the enactment of the PHC professional ethos is facilitated by structural factors. For example, family doctors were allocated a specific time slot, about one day per week, for clinical research and they usually have more time per patient than hospital oncologists. This invites us to consider medical paternalism in a more nuanced way, particularly in the context of sever diseases such as cancer, as intrinsic to the asymmetry that defines any relation of care (Livingston, 2012, 164–166). Thus, the way Dr Flora's performs community engagement is not neutralizing the asymmetry of care, but is clearly challenging the paternalism that prevails in Cuban oncology by adapting care to each situation and facilitating interactions between cancer patients and the wider community.

From 'chronic' to palliative treatments: engaging to ensure continuity of cancer care

Chronic diseases affect people throughout their life through periods of stability, acute crisis and slow deterioration, which requires constant adjustments of treatments and relations with their social worlds (Strauss, 1975). In the context of cancer, a usually lethal disease, Baszanger (2012) shows how chronicity is shaped by multiple, uncertain and often invasive interventions that constantly redefine the frontier between curative and palliative care. In the recent trend towards chronic disease management in global health, Whitmarsh (2013) argues that compliance is a central feature, which consists in disciplining patients in order to adapt to new therapeutic regimens. In the context of the Cuban PHC clinical trial, I show how PHC practitioners are enacting community engagement to adapt biomedicine to people's needs, and, by doing so, ensure continuity of care from chronic treatment to palliative care.

My ethnography shows how PHC professionals are adjusting or even bypassing the clinical trial's protocol to address specific demands linked to a chronic cancer management. When the patient could not come to the consultation, because of his/her deteriorating state or because his close relatives were temporarily unable to transport him/her, the family doctors agree to delay the treatment. Furthermore, in the interviews, many family doctors and nurses mentioned that they 'vaccinated' patients' at the *consultorio*, or even at their home. Other types of adjustments were related to the reduction of the frequency of immunizations because of chronic pain in the injection sites. Reported to clinical trial manager as 'small protocol deviations' since they were planned by the trial, such adaptations were usually coordinated with the hospital oncologist. These practices highlight how PHC professionals adapt care to the specificities of chronic disease temporalities. Thus, they conduct activities that are typical to their professional ethos, such as at-home visits and educational activity.

Lisa, a nurse in an Eastern province, decided to set up 'educative speeches' (*charlas educativas*) at the polyclinic for patients, their relatives, and neighbours interested in the themes of the talks. She told me that for her: 'the clinical trial is not just about the vaccine but is also a community activity'. The main goal of the educative speeches is to inform patients and their relatives about the risk to which chronic lung cancer patients are particularly vulnerable at home: dust, and smoking (that can exacerbate respiratory failure), but also diseases transmitted by mosquitoes (that can easily kill immune-deficient persons). While these educative sessions coincide with both the mass-mobilization and the current global health framework of educational health designed to discipline behaviours of chronic patients (Feinsilver, 1993; Whitmarsh, 2013), they also create a space where lung cancer patients can interact with other members of the community. In effect, some sessions are dedicated to lung cancer, and patients are invited to provide testimonies of their disease experiences. Furthermore, Lisa joyfully mentioned me that the local PHC research team organizes 'vaccination birthday parties' at the polyclinic, when patients reached one year of survival in the clinical trial.

Lisa's case shows how the form of community engagement that PHC practitioners preform through activities goes beyond the clinical trial's implementation to meet chronic cancer patients' needs. They also pursue engagement when patients are withdrawn from the protocol due to deteriorating health status. Most family doctors and nurses I interviewed told me that when the patient is withdrawn from the protocol, they accompany him or her until their final days, even if it is not part of the task of the PHC research team. As it is planned by the health system, it should be the *consultorio's* team that should provide palliative care to the cancer patient with some support provided by polyclinics' and hospitals' specialists (Figueredo Villa, 2011). Yet, as the *consultorio* team is generally not trained to follow terminal cancer patients, and overwhelmed by other activities, patients must go to the hospitals, where there is no specific structure for palliative care. Thus, by accompanying patients beyond the protocol, the PHC professionals involved in the clinical trial create a continuity of care from chronic treatment to palliative care through engagement.

Conclusion

In this paper, I have attempted to capture the forms of community engagement in a PHC oncology clinical trials taking place in contemporary Cuba's socialist biomedicine. Although community engagement is not a formal component of the clinical research programme, I have shown how it is performed as part of the PHC professional ethos as an implicit practice enacted by family doctors and nurses through local initiatives at the polyclinic level. By engaging communities in the course of the trial, PHC practitioners build an emerging form of community cancer care in a context of prevailing paternalism within Cuban oncology that provides both moral and political dimensions of care (Livingston, 2012). Thus, my findings extends Gibbon's argument (2013), that PHC professionals are conferring another meaning to Cuban state socialism, as a biopolitical regime not only based on paternalism and egalitarian delivery of social goods (as in the mass mobilization model), but also on individual and communities' capacities to reshape and transform health politics.

To some extent, the form of community engagement I have explored overlaps with existing practices within global health research projects. As historians of scientific and medical relations during the Cold War era argued (Geltzer, 2012; Vargha, 2014), it is crucial to avoid reproducing essentialized oppositions between socialist and capitalist societies. As showcased in Dr Flora 'small corner', the family doctor is attempting to reconcile the biomedical autonomous subject with more collective forms of personhood, a stake described in other Global Health contexts (Sariola & Simpson, 2011). Bioethical approaches on informed consent attempt to take into account these local conceptions of individual and collective ethics (Lavery et al., 2010). Lisa's 'educative speeches' can also be related to 'community activities' designed to provide 'information' promoted by global health projects (*Ibid.*). However, I have argued that the form of community engagement taking place in Cuban socialist biomedicine is alternative to global health's dominant paradigm because it builds upon and strengthens existing infrastructures of public health. It is not undertaken as a bounded set of activities disarticulated from local health research and local public service delivery as is frequent in global health interventions (Biehl & Petryna, 2013; Crane, 2013; Pfeiffer, 2003). When PHC practitioners practice community engagement to promote patients' self-affirmation, they reproduce the state idea that family doctors and nurses are among the actors most entitled to represent communities' interests. When Dr Maria is making the cancer treatment understandable to patients by echoing prophylactic vaccination, she is creating continuity between state dedication to eradicate infectious diseases and its commitment to offer innovative cancer treatment at the level of PHC. Even if Dr Flora built her *huequito* in the polyclinic's backyard because there was no adapted consultation room available in her polyclinic, she created a cancer consultation place open to other people in the neighbourhood. While global health research projects frequently produce 'material artefacts' that will not last after the intervention (Kelly, 2011; Montgomery, 2017), PHC professionals are performing community engagement to integrate oncology innovation to the PHC infrastructures and the local ethos of care. Thus, they are contributing to building a new form of cancer ambulatory treatment that integrates chronic treatment and palliative care. Given the still emerging trend toward chronic diseases in global health (Livingston, 2012; Whitmarsh, 2013), the Cuban experience in PHC cancer clinical trials offers a novel perspective on community engagement in the field of oncology, one that constantly attempts to adapt the biomedical machinery to both existing public health infrastructures and people's needs.

Notes

1. All acronyms for Cuban institutions are in Spanish.
2. Among others, this includes the Committees for the Defence of the Revolution (CDR), the labour syndicates or the Federation of Cuban women.
3. In 2014, there were 11'550 *consultorios*, 451 polyclinics and 152 hospitals on the island (Minsap, 2014).
4. All the names are pseudonyms, yet reflecting gender.
5. Cuba has one of the largest vaccination programs in the world, covering against 13 diseases (see Lage, 2008).

Disclosure statement

The author reports no conflicts of interest.

Funding

This work was supported by the Institut Francilien Recherche Innovation Société (IFRIS) [Mobility grant]; Institut National Du Cancer (INCa) [PhD scholarship]

References

Adams, V., Burke, N. J., & Whitmarsh, I. (2014). Slow research: Thoughts for a movement in global health. *Medical Anthropology, 33*(3), 179–197.

Andaya, E. (2009). The gift of health: Socialist medical practice and shifting material and moral economies in post-Soviet Cuba. *Medical Anthropology Quarterly, 23*(4), 357–374.

Atlani-Duault, L. (2008). *Humanitarian aid in post-Soviet countries: An anthropological perspective*. London: Routledge.

Baszanger, I. (2012). One more chemo or one too many? Defining the limits of treatment and innovation in medical oncology. *Social Science & Medicine (1982), 75*(5), 864–872.

Batista Moliner, R., & González Ochoa, E. (2000). Evaluación de la vigilancia en la atención primaria de salud: Una propuesta metodológica [Evaluation of surveillance in primary healthcare: A methodological proposition]. *Revista Cubana de Medicina Tropical, 52*(1), 55–65.

Beldarraín, E. (2013). Poliomyelitis and its elimination in Cuba: An historical overview. *MEDICC Review, 15*(2), 30–36.

Biehl, J., & Petryna, A. (2013). *When people come first: Critical studies in global health.* Princeton, NJ: Princeton University Press.

Birn, A.-E. (2014). Philanthrocapitalism, past and present: The Rockefeller Foundation, the Gates Foundation, and the setting(s) of the international/global health agenda. *Hypothesis, 12*(1), Retrieved from Hypothesis Journal Website http://www.hypothesisjournal.com/wp-content/uploads/2014/11/HJ229%E2%80%94FIN_Nov1_2014.pdf

Brotherton, P. S. (2012). *Revolutionary medicine: Health and the Body in Post-soviet Cuba.* Durham: Duke University Press.

Brown, T. M., Cueto, M., & Fee, E. (2006). The World Health Organization and the transition from 'international' to 'global' public health. *American Journal of Public Health, 96*(1), 62–72.

Burke, N. (2013). *Health travels: Cuban health(care) on and off the Island.* San Francisco, CA: University of California Medical Humanities Press.

Crane, J. T. (2013). *Scrambling for Africa: AIDS, expertise, and the rise of American global health science.* Ithaca, NY: Cornell University Press.

Davis, C., & Abraham, J. (2011). Desperately seeking cancer drugs: Explaining the emergence and outcomes of accelerated pharmaceutical regulation. *Sociology of Health & Illness, 33*(5), 731–747.

Fassin, D. (2008). The elementary forms of care: An empirical approach to ethics in a South African Hospital. *Social Science & Medicine (1982), 67*(2), 262–270.

Feinsilver, J. M. (1993). *Healing the masses: Cuban health politics at home and abroad.* Berkeley, CA: University of California Press.

Figueredo Villa, K. (2011). Cuidados paliativos: Evolución y desarrollo en Cuba [Palliative care: evolution and development in Cuba]. *Enfermería Global, 10*(21), 1–10.

Geltzer, A. (2012). In a distorted mirror: The cold war and U.S.-Soviet biomedical cooperation and (Mis)understanding, 1956–1977. *Journal of Cold War Studies, 14*(3), 39–63.

Gibbon, S. (2011). Family medicine, 'La Herencia' and breast cancer; understanding the (dis)continuities of predictive genetics in Cuba. *Social Science & Medicine (1982), 72*(11), 1784.

Gibbon, S. E. (2013). Science, sentiment, and the state: Community genetics and pursuit of public health in Cuba. *Medical Anthropology Quarterly, 27*(4), 531–549.

Graber, N. (2013). Les activités d'un réseau d'ONG à Cuba: Internationalisme médical et santé globale [The activities of a NGO network in Cuba: Medical internationalism and global health]. *Revue Tiers Monde, 215*, 149–164.

Janes, C. R., & Corbett, K. K. (2009). Anthropology and global health. *Annual Review of Anthropology, 38*(1), 167–183.

Kelly, A. (2011). Pragmatic fact-making: Contracts and contexts in the UK and the Gambia. In C. Will & T. Moreira (Eds.), *Medical proofs, social experiments: Clinical trials in shifting contexts* (pp. 121–137). Farnham: Ashgate.

Keshavjee, S. (2014). *Blind spot: How neoliberalism infiltrated global health* (Vols. 1–1). Oakland, CA: University of California press.

King, K. F., Kolopack, P., Merritt, M. W., & Lavery, J. V. (2014). Community engagement and the human infrastructure of global health research. *BMC Medical Ethics, 15*, 816.

Koch, E. (2013). *Free market tuberculosis: Managing epidemics in post-Soviet Georgia.* Nashville: Vanderbilt University Press.

Lage, A. (2008). Connecting immunology research to public health: Cuban biotechnology. *Nature Immunology, 9*(2), 109–112.

Lage, A., & Crombet, T. (2011). Control of advanced cancer: The road to chronicity. *International Journal of Environmental Research and Public Health, 8*(12), 683–697.

Lakoff, A. (2010). Two regimes of global health. *Humanity: An International Journal of Human Rights, Humanitarianism, and Development, 1*(1), 59–79.

Lavery, J. V., Tinadana, P. O., Scott, T. W., Harrington, L. C., Ramsey, J. M., Ytuarte-Nuñez, C., & James, A. A. (2010). Towards a framework for community engagement in global health research. *Trends in Parasitology, 26*(6), 279–283.

Livingston, J. (2012). *Improvising medicine: An African oncology ward in an emerging cancer epidemic.* Duke University Press.

MacQueen, K. M., Bhan, A., Frohlich, J., Holzer, J., & Sugarman, J. (2015). Evaluating community engagement in global health research: The need for metrics. *BMC Medical Ethics, 16*, 1380.

Minsap. (2014), Anuario Estadístico del Ministerio de Salud Pública [Annual statistics from the Ministry of Public Health]. Retrieved from the Infomed Website http://www.bvscuba.sld.cu/2017/11/20/anuario-estadistico-de-salud-de-cuba/

Mol, A., Moser, I., & Pols, J. (Eds.). (2010). *Care in practice: On tinkering in clinics, homes and farms* (Vols. 1–1). Bielefeld: Transcript.

Montgomery, C. M. (2017). Clinical trials and the drive to material standardisation. *Science & Technology Studies, 30*(4), 30–44.

Pfeiffer, J. (2003). International NGOs and primary health care in Mozambique: The need for a new model of collaboration. *Social Science & Medicine, 56*(4), 725–738.

Pfeiffer, J., & Chapman, R. (2010). Anthropological perspectives on structural adjustment and public health. *Annual Review of Anthropology, 39*(1), 149–165.

Prince, R. J. & Marsland, R. (Eds.). (2014). *Making and unmaking public health in Africa: Ethnographic and historical perspectives.* Athens: Ohio University Press.

Reed, G. (2008). Cuba's primary health care revolution: 30 Years on. *Bulletin of the World Health Organization, 86*(5), 327–329.

Reid-Henry, S. M. (2010). *The Cuban cure: Reason and resistance in global science.* Chicago, IL: University of Chicago Press.

Romero, T. (2009). Changing the paradigm of cancer control in cuba. *MEDICC Review, 11*(3), 5–7.

Sanchez, L., Perez, D., Cruz, G., Castro, M., Kourí, G., Shkedy, Z., & Van der Stuyft, P. (2009). Intersectoral coordination, community empowerment and dengue prevention: Six years of controlled interventions in Playa Municipality, Havana, Cuba. *Tropical Medicine & International Health: TM & IH, 14*(11), 1356–1364.

Sariola, S. & Simpson, B. (2011). Theorising the 'human subject' in biomedical research: International clinical trials and bioethics discourses in contemporary Sri Lanka. *Social Science & Medicine, 73*(4), 515–521.

Spiegel, J. M., & Yassi, A. (2004). Lessons from the margins of globalization: Appreciating the Cuban health paradox. *Journal of Public Health Policy, 25*(1), 85–110.

Strauss, A. L. (1975). *Chronic illness and the quality of life.* Saint Louis, MO: Mosby.

Vargha, D. (2014). Between East and West: Polio vaccination across the iron curtain in cold war hungary. *Bulletin of the History of Medicine, 88*(2), 319–342.

Wailoo, K., Livingston, J., Epstein, S., & Aronowitz, R. (2010). *Three shots at prevention: The HPV vaccine and the politics of medicine's simple solutions.* Baltimore, CA: JHU Press.

Whitmarsh, I. (2013). The turn to chronic diseases in global health. In J. Biehl & A. Petryna (Eds.), *When people come first: Critical studies in global health* (pp. 320–324). Princeton, NJ: Princeton University Press.

WHO. (1975). *Health by the people.* Geneva: WHO.

Who is 'in' and who is 'out'? Participation of older persons in health research and the interplay between capital, habitus and field

Lieke Oldenhof ⓘD and Rik Wehrens

ABSTRACT

Inclusion and exclusion processes in community engagement do not take place in a vacuum, but are embedded in social, political and institutional contexts. To better capture the interplay between the individual agency of community participants and organizational structures in health research, we use a Bourdieusian framework. The notions of capital, habitus and field allow us to analyse how inclusion and exclusion of older persons in a Dutch healthcare research- and improvement programme are processually shaped overtime. The findings demonstrate that due to the influence of the medical and policy field, older persons with social, cultural and symbolic capital were included in target group panels. Frail older persons lacking these types of capital were often excluded. Despite the high amount of capital, the formally 'included' participants still experienced difficulties in engaging effectively in a medical research setting. We distinguish various strategies that older persons developed during the course of the programme to deal with this problem: (1) professionalization, (2) responsibilization, (3) pluralization, (4) opting out. Using these strategies older participants were able to incrementally change the medical field by shifting the focus to quality of life and welfare. We conclude that it is by definition impossible to 'exclude exclusion' at the start of care improvement programmes. It is only in the many pragmatic and mundane choices of 'doing participation' that more inclusive engagement can be realized.

Introduction

Community engagement has developed into a widespread policy ideal that is viewed as intrinsically good as it promises democratic decision-making, empowerment and legitimacy (Bensing, 2000; Boote, Telford, & Cooper, 2002; Hanley, Truesdale, King, Elbourne, & Chalmers, 2001; Van de Bovenkamp, Trappenburg, & Grit, 2009). This ideal has been translated into various formats and governance structures, such as patient councils, community membership of ethics committees and funding boards (Van de Bovenkamp et al., 2009). Also in global health research, efforts to promote community engagement in the design and evaluation of research have increased in the past decade (Lavery et al., 2010). Despite the inclusive promise of engagement, however, risks of community exploitation and exclusion of patient perspectives are still pervasive (Gbadegesin & Wendler, 2006). The literature offers different explanations for the gap between policy ideal and practice as well as solutions to close this gap. Studies on health literacy focus on the lack of individual capacities to effectively process health information leading to exclusion of patients in decision-making (Nutbeam, 2008; Ratzan, 2001). Perceived solutions are strengthening skills and capacities via education to make patients and communities more 'health literate'. Global health researchers have developed guidelines for effective community participation, emphasizing the need for trust building, ownership by the community and co-production of knowledge (Lavery et al., 2010). In addition, organizational literature provides useful insights into specific facilitators and barriers that enable or limit inclusive participation (e.g. staff capacity, financial resources and accountability requirements) (Légaré, Ratté, Gravel, & Graham, 2008; Luxford, Safran, & Delbanco, 2011; Montori, Gafni, & Charles, 2006).

Although these bodies of literature offer valuable explanations and solutions for reducing the gap between the policy ideal of community engagement and practice, we argue that there is still too little attention for a more detailed analysis of the interplay between individual agency and organizational structures in how inclusion and exclusion are shaped in mundane practices. Engagement does not take place in a social vacuum, but is embedded in particular social, political and institutional contexts (King, Kolopack, Merritt, & Lavery, 2014). To better capture this dynamic interplay, we use the Bourdieusian framework of capital, habitus and field to analyse how inclusion and exclusion are processually shaped. This framework makes visible the relations between institutional context, embedded work routines and individual decisions of actors. Additionally, we use the concept of 'micro-advantages' (Gengler, 2014) to show how the mobilization of capital can result in subtle advantages vis-à-vis other participating actors.

We analyse a Dutch case of target group participation in the National Program of Elderly Care (NPEC). This programme aims to improve the quality of care for frail older persons with multiple conditions by the development of (1) regional networks for care and research, in which target group panels (consisting of older persons) were positioned as important network partners; (2) transition experiments and research projects to improve the quality of care; (3) the implementation of new interventions in medical care and public health. In each, older persons were actively encouraged to participate in the evaluation, design and implementation of research and interventions.

This empirical case is interesting for several reasons. First, older persons that participated in panels were generally well-educated with much managerial experience. Despite their privileged background and formal inclusion, they still experienced difficulties in effectively participating in the evaluation and design of research. From the perspective of health literacy, we cannot explain why literate older persons still faced such difficulties and sometimes felt socially excluded from decision-making despite being formally included. Second, the organizational conditions to enhance participation of older persons were ideal on paper. The NPEC was positioned as a unique programme in making participation of older persons a funding requirement for research proposals and network development. Despite these important organizational facilitators, there was a continuous struggle of participation between medical researchers and target group panels.

Our analysis provides insights in how inclusion and exclusion processes are shaped by the interplay between individual agency and organizational structures. In the discussion, we will reflect on the implications of our analysis for the ethics and politics of community engagement in global health. First, however, we explain the concepts of capital, habitus, field and micro-advantages, showing the relevance of a Bourdieusian framework in studying participation.

A Bourdieusian approach: capital, field and habitus

The work of Bourdieu is influential in sociology, but also applied productively in different health-related contexts as various as the relation between dog-ownership and walking (Degeling, Rock, Rogers, & Riley, 2016); drug use (Van Hout, 2011); vulnerabilities of marginalized sex workers (Stoebenau, 2009), patient-provider interactions (Dubbin, Chang, & Shim, 2013) and infection control (Brown, Crawford, Nerlich, & Koteyko, 2008). These studies explore relationships between individual experiences, social interactions and the institutional environment.

The concepts of field, capital and habitus are conceptual tools to understand stratification processes in social spaces (Bourdieu, 1990). Bourdieu conceptualizes society as a plurality of social fields (Siisiäinen, 2003), described as 'a series of structures, institutions, authorities and activities, all of which relate to the people acting within the field' (Rhynas, 2005, p. 181). Fields incrementally change overtime due to power dynamics that can challenge the boundaries of the field (Rhynas, 2005). Actors are considered to be simultaneously *embedded within* fields and at the same time struggle with and change these fields. Separate fields (e.g. science, medicine, politics, education) have furthermore developed their own distinctive institutional dynamics (Brown et al., 2008).

In order to obtain influence and status in a certain field, people need to mobilize capital. Bourdieu views the value of capital as context-specific: it is appreciated differently depending on the field (Bourdieu, 1990). He distinguishes various types of capital, including social capital (networks and relations), cultural capital (education and skills), financial capital (property and other resources) and symbolic capital (prestige). These forms of capital are convertible (Portes, 2000). Bourdieu originally defined social capital as 'the aggregate of the actual or potential resources which are linked to possession of a durable network of more or less institutionalized relationships of mutual acquaintance or recognition' (Bourdieu, 1985, p. 248, cited in Portes, 1998). Social capital is thus the goodwill available to individuals or groups, arising from the structure and content of someone's social relations (Adler & Kwon, 2002).

Cultural and symbolic capital are other forms of capital. Cultural capital consists of long-lasting dispositions, educational qualifications and knowledge of cultural goods (Bourdieu, 1990). It includes informal education transmitted through the family, political parties and cultural groups, but also formal education. Symbolic capital involves the attribution of prestige and credit. It includes not only displays of social standing, but also the collective judgements that shape how these displays are perceived and the consequences of such attributions (e.g. marks of recognition) (Bourdieu & Wacquant, 2013). Together these various forms of capital add up to an individual's overall capital.

In between field and capital, Bourdieu positioned the 'habitus', denoting lasting dispositions that are unconsciously embodied and internalized, thereby guiding how we collectively think and act (Bourdieu, 1990). The habitus is not only social, but also a taken-for-granted embodied reality (Rhynas, 2005). It not merely passively reproduces dominant ideology, but functions as a generative principle (Brown et al., 2008). It is durable overtime, and although its structures can be modified, this is typically a slow, accumulative process (Siisiäinen, 2003). Habitus can thus be viewed as a system of embodied dispositions that organizes the ways in which individuals perceive the social world around them and react to it. As dispositions are usually shared by people with similar backgrounds, members with a long history in a particular field have more time to internalize the socialized norms and tendencies that make-up a person's habitus (e.g. doctors).

Although Bourdieu's earlier work is criticized for its overdeterministic emphasis on structures, his later work focuses more explicitly on agency and institutional change (cf. Reay, 2004). Therefore, Bourdieu's theoretical apparatus enables a detailed analysis of how specific actors mobilize various forms of capital and interact with the routines that make-up the broader institutional field.

Bourdieu's framework offers an analytical lense to understand inclusion and exclusion processes in the participation of older persons for three reasons. First, the combined concepts of social, cultural and symbolic capital are crucial for understanding not only how some actors are able to achieve advantages, but also how others are excluded from participation and its potential benefits (Bourdieu, 1990; Gengler, 2014; Shim, 2010). Capital can also be used to constrain opportunities to non-network members, leading to disadvantages for other actors (Adler & Kwon, 2002; Portes, 1998). Second, 'engagement does not happen entirely *de novo* and the healthcare field is not just plastic to the participants' will: it imposes limits' (Brown et al., 2008, p. 1048). This implies that studies focusing on individual capacities overlook the interplay between individual agency (used here in its everyday meaning of the ability to act and make choices) and organizational structures that shape inclusion and exclusion. The notion of habitus is better able to address this interplay between agency and structures in how people negotiate change as the concept recognizes both the role of dispositions and structures that people have internalized through socialization *and* the opportunities for change (as habitus constrains but does not fully determine thought and action). Third, the concepts are valuable for explaining differences in benefits gained from mobilizing capital. These benefits are sometimes described in terms of 'micro-advantages', denoting small gains which incrementally can lead to the acquisition of significant (health) improvements (Gengler, 2014; Shim, 2010).

Based on this theoretical framework, this paper investigates the following question: How is the inclusion and exclusion of older persons in the NPEC processually shaped through the interplay between individual agency and organizational structures?

Methods

Our analysis is based on qualitative research of the National Program of Elderly Care (NPEC) that took place between 2008 and 2016. With a total budget of over 80 million euros, it was one of the largest care improvement programmes in the Netherlands. The NPEC is funded through the Ministry of Health, Welfare and Sports, who commissioned the Netherlands Organisation for Health Research and Development (a large funding body for health research and innovation) to further develop and monitor the programme. In the development of the programme, a national programme committee – responsible for the operational governance – was established by the funding body. Members of this committee had a high public profile and were viewed as experts in research, policy and healthcare.

As researchers, we were commissioned by the Netherlands Organisation for Health Research and Development to evaluate the NPEC. In this role, we conducted 53 semi-structured interviews with 63 respondents, ranging from 50 to 150 minutes per interview, 90 minutes average. We interviewed different stakeholders, including older persons of the target group panels and national representatives of elderly associations ($n = 21$). We also interviewed medical researchers and representatives of medical associations, national policy-makers at the Ministry of Health, Welfare and Sports and the funding body, network coordinators and other stakeholders. The interviews with older persons focused on the participants' backgrounds, their experiences with evaluating/monitoring research projects, the workload of participating, required skills and their interactions with researchers. To supplement the interview data, we conducted observations of meetings of the target group panels and analysed relevant documents pertaining to target group participation.

All interviews were transcribed verbatim. For the analysis, we used social, cultural and symbolic capital, habitus, field and micro-advantages as 'sensitizing concepts' (Blumer, 1954). Key themes that inductively emerged from the analysis were the ways inclusion and exclusion was shaped, the different strategies older participants developed to deal with participation in a predominantly medical domain, and the consequences of these strategies.

Results

The organization of the programme and the selection of participants

The goal of the NPEC was to improve care for 'frail older persons', operationalized in terms of older persons having multiple mental and/or physical problems (e.g. medical diseases, housing problems and loneliness). To achieve this goal, more scientific substantiation of effective interventions and evidence-based methods was considered to be necessary by the funding body (ZonMw, 2008). To shape the research required for this, regional networks ($n = 9$) were developed in which University Medical Centres (UMCs) were appointed as network leaders that invited other public service organizations (e.g. in care and well-being) to join. Important aims of the regional networks were integration of service provision for frail older persons, promotion of target group participation, research and the implementation of interventions as diverse as integrated care pathways, screening instruments for frailty and neighbourhood community engagement.

An important emancipatory ideal of the funding body was to give frail older persons 'voice' and 'choice' in the design, evaluation and monitoring of research. Although there were no strict criteria for 'successful engagement', the programme documentation highlights that the funding body saw active involvement of older persons as important *means* for developing more relevant research that better fits the needs of this group. The final programme document explicitly mentions the consultation of target group panels as an important requirement for the regional networks' eligibility for funding (ZonMw, 2008).

To meet this requirement, the UMC's took the lead in setting-up target group panels and recruiting participants for these panels. The participants had a professional history in various domains, including social work, politics, labour unions and private companies. Additionally, some informal caregivers also participated in target group panels. The age range of participants was between 55 and 90 years.[1] The number of participants of target group panels varied from $n = 8$ to $n = 15$. The general number of active participants in all target group panels and governance boards of regional networks gradually increased to $n = 175$. Ethnic minorities were severely underrepresented in this number.[2]

Although the goal of the NPEC was formulated in terms of care improvement for frail older persons, in practice *frail* older persons were largely excluded from participation in target group panels, whereas relatively 'resilient' older persons in terms of health status and social-economic background were over-represented. This selection of relatively resilient older persons was highly structured by the medical and policy field in which the programme was developed. Although many respondents argued that the UMC's medical focus did not align with the broader focus on well-being that mattered for older persons, they were nevertheless made responsible for the development of the regional networks and, therefore, also for the set-up of target group panels. The UMC's leading role can be explained in terms of the strongly established medical field they are part of and the strong social, cultural and symbolic capital that flows from this.

Described above as 'a series of structures, institutions, authorities and activities' (Rhynas, 2005, p. 181), the UMCs are key institutions and have a strong, historically developed, authoritative position in medicine. Supported by a strong umbrella organization to coordinate efforts and negotiate with policy-makers, the UMCs have become important institutions in the medical field. Many actors also developed the cultural capital to write research proposals that matched the criteria and the more implicit demands (correct language and terminology) of the funding body. The field of welfare, on the other hand, was much more fragmented and did not have a strong umbrella organization. Furthermore, many actors in this field lacked the cultural capital to quickly produce research proposals that met the formal and informal criteria of the funding body. These aspects help explain why the UMCs 'took the lead' in the regional networks, which consequentially shaped the selection of particular older participants for the panels (i.e. those who had acquired some forms of capital, see below) (Interview with member of the programme committee, representative of the mental care domain, male).

The influence of the policy field becomes visible in the time pressure the UMCs experienced at the start of the NPEC to set-up the required target group panels, as a result of the predominant logic in this field: the logic that policy programmes run for four years and that a certain percentage of the budget needs to be attributed in the first year.[3] Therefore, many research calls were organized in the first year, placing the networks under heavy time pressure. Consequentially, UMCs often pragmatically selected older persons from their own personal networks (e.g. retired university lecturers) or through professional patient platforms. Thus, especially older persons with a large amount of social capital were selected for the panels. This social capital could consist of an established network with medical researchers through previous work experience or of a network established by other means (elderly associations, unions or political/managerial experience). Although these forms of social capital do not necessarily provide expertise in reviewing research proposals nor presuppose health literacy, they were appreciated by medical researchers as important qualities for participation.

Despite the importance of capital for *inclusion* in target group panels, exclusion of frail older persons in those panels cannot solely be explained by a lack of capital. Significantly, the format of participating in committee meetings and panels also seems to preclude a part of the target group of frail older persons. Problems of physical access to meeting locations and the need to travel across the country also played an important role in shaping formal exclusion. People having difficulties following conversations due to their condition were also less likely to be able to participate.

Experimenting with participation of older persons

The analysis above showed the influence of established fields (medical and policy) on how participation of older persons was shaped in the beginning of the programme, leading to the inclusion of persons with specific forms of social capital and the exclusion of persons lacking this capital. Processes of inclusion and exclusion are not static, however, and continued to be shaped in the course of the programme through the interplay between the various forms of capital, habitus and field.

In the early days of the programme, medical researchers had particular ideas about what constitutes a 'good' participant. Older persons with executive networks (social capital) and high education (cultural capital) were valued as legitimate actors in the medical field because they were viewed as more effective (Interview with medical researcher, female). At the same time, the experiences of older persons were often discredited because they were expressed in a style that made generalization hard (several respondents talked about the '$N = 1$ elderly' in this case). A programme committee member expresses her difficulties with the way in which older persons often expressed their experiences:

> I deeply respect those professors for their patience, because sometimes it drives you mad!

> *What aspects drove you mad?*

> Well, if as a researcher you ask older persons: what do you think is important? Well, ok: 'the mother of my granddad has this and this', you know what it's like, that's the way you talk with your neighbour on the birthday of your sister. But you need to be able to look beyond your own casuistry. The ones that can do this are the older persons that have studied more. And when you haven't (studied) you get stuck in your own casuistry. They also raise good points, but well, the *energy* that you have to put into it … (Interview with former coordinator NPEC, policy maker, female)

This quote shows that individual experiences of older persons are not immediately considered valuable in the medical field; they require much additional work that is not appreciated.

Older participants were thus implicitly expected to make the 'right' kinds of argument, which means seeing the bigger picture and refraining from 'nit-picking' (Interview with medical researcher, female). In terms of cultural capital, older persons were required to be knowledgeable about the 'appropriate' conversational and argumentative style (to argue beyond individual cases). Older persons that have acquired this cultural capital are valued more by medical researchers, consequentially increasing their symbolic capital as well.

These examples point to how older persons learn to become active members by following the rules of engagement. Such rules of engagement turn out to be hard to change. They have a long history in the way the funding body facilitates and organizes participation of target groups and they also fit in the Dutch deliberative policy tradition. The notions of habitus and field thus help explain why participation is organized in this deliberative manner: the rules of engagement for participation have obtained a kind of obduracy that is the result of a Dutch policy tradition and bureaucratic ways of working that have historically developed and have become both institutionalized in procedures and routines and internalized by many persons as socialized norms about how deliberation should be organized.

Even older persons with much social and cultural capital had difficulties in participating in such settings, because of different customs in the medical field and institutional barriers in the policy field. First, they emphasized the inaccessibility of scientific terminology:

> [The projects] have to lead to improvement of elderly care. That perspective is indeed included, but it remained very far removed from (older persons). […] The terminology …. I am no pussycat, but you almost need to have a dictionary at your disposal. Jargon! (Interview with member of elderly advocacy group, male)

The use of scientific jargon makes it more difficult for many older persons to participate effectively in panels. This jargon is not only part of the 'rules' of the medical field (as specific terms and criteria for research apply, including medical terminology and methodological precision), but also closely tied to the policy field, where the established procedure is to find scientific experts for peer reviewing the content of the proposals without necessarily taking into account the lay criteria through which older persons define good research (such as relevance and the link between medical care and welfare).

A second difficulty is the narrow time schedule in which many projects had to be developed. Target group panels were only involved in the evaluation of research proposals that were almost finished with the submission deadline approaching fast. This made dissenting opinions less likely:

> There is enormous time pressure on those meetings, so if you take a formalistic stance you only frustrate the discussion (Interview with former member of target group panel, male)

This quote shows that although *formally* target group panels were considered important for judging the proposals, established work routines in the medical field, in combination with the limited symbolic capital of older persons in relation to medical researchers, made it hard, if not impossible, in this stage for older persons to 'keep their foot down' (i.e. taking a 'formalistic stance').

A major consequence of these difficulties was that representatives in target group panels increasingly experienced that their perspective was used instrumentally. A respondent vividly recalls his frustration vented during one of the meetings:

> Where did all the money go in the first two years (of NPEC)? I said that in 2010. The bomb exploded.

> *How did people respond to what you said?*

> Dead quiet. I said in a loud voice: 'We are not here to promote people with a university degree to doctor, we are here for older persons'. Quiet. Very quiet it became. Then someone responded: 'you are right X'. (…). At a certain moment I said: 'give us the opportunity to think for ourselves and take charge for once. Of course, we have ideas ourselves, we are here for a reason! (Interview with member of target group panel, male)

This frustration was experienced by more participants. Feelings of exclusion were further strengthened because research proposals initiated bottom-up by target group panels were often not funded by the funding body, that used scientific evaluation criteria to assess the worth of proposals (see above). Formal criteria for receiving funding conflicted here with the 'lay' perspective of target group panels.

In sum, the medical and policy field turned out to be hard to change without the necessary cultural capital (e.g. procedural knowledge about how regular procedures work and how 'normal' research proposals should be written and evaluated).

Strategies to participate in the medical field

Although the analysis thus far seems to point out that the 'voice' of older participants was limited and that the older persons involved in the panels were not able to destabilize existing power relations, such a conclusion would be too bleak. During the course of the programme, we saw that the voice of community members gradually led to substantive changes. The programme committee and the funding body became increasingly aware of the frustrations of target group panels and the shortcomings of this particular form of engagement. They did not significantly alter the structure of engagement, but they did support target group panels by organizing theme-based conferences about engagement and by more tailored funding opportunities.

Target group panels themselves also developed responses to the difficulties they experienced. We distinguish four strategies. Some of these strategies highlight how older persons have internalized some of the tacit rules of the medical field as part of their habitus, whereas other strategies show older persons ignoring or attempting to change the status quo. To strengthen the position of the target group panels and counterbalance the dominance of the medical field, *professionalization* of older persons was a frequently used strategy. Professionalization entailed the coaching of target group representatives in order to develop the 'right' cultural capital to participate in the medical field. This strategy was also supported by the programme committee of the NPEC, who initiated a specific project called 'Powerful Client Perspective'. This project aimed to strengthen the voice of older persons and included various training sessions for target group panels, in order to learn how to lobby and effectively frame talking points during meetings with medical researchers. Additionally, the umbrella organization for elderly associations wrote a handbook on 'how to' participate for the community of older persons.

Although professionalization can strengthen the lay perspective vis-à-vis the medical perspective through the enhancement of participants' cultural capital (both formal, through the trainings, and informal, through peer discussions), this strategy still takes the medical field as a starting point. In some occasions, this led to the well-known risk of 'proto-professionalization' (De Swaan, 1988; Dent, 2006) when target group panels adopted scientific jargon and selected 'professional' candidates for target group panels:

> A: Tomorrow I have an interview with someone who wants to become member. That person has a wonderful CV. Since I became chair (of the target group panel) I say: 'before we hire someone, I want a CV. It doesn't have to be 3 pages, 1 page will do' (…)
>
> B: We put that on paper beforehand: what are the criteria that a member of the target group panel will have to meet?
>
> *What are the criteria?*
>
> B: uh well, at a minimum you need to be able to talk well, to have executive experience, to be able to think in policy terms, have a network, those kind of elements.
>
> A: and you need to be involved. These are more or less 8 criteria that we have listed. Those are the things we are looking for (Interview with two members of target group panel, male and female).

This quote shows how professionalized target group panels were complicit in the further exclusion of older persons with little social and cultural capital.

A second strategy is *responsibilization*. This refers to a governing technique to mould responsible citizens who then internalize certain duties and govern themselves accordingly (Dean, 1999). Through their long-time participation in the NPEC, some older persons seemed to have internalized the tacit rules of the medical field as part of their habitus through their continuous socialization into the field-specific rules. This resulted in a heightened sense of responsibility of older persons who have internalized their participatory duties. Responsibilization became manifest in how target group panels deal with 'participatory work'. This includes carefully reading all minutes from previous meetings, dividing tasks into different 'work groups', 'doing your homework' (some older persons came with large stacks of notes to the meetings) and in general being 'well-prepared'. This requires much time: some respondents emphasized that they spent up to 30 hours per week. A second example of responsibilization is the corrective behaviour between peers. Members of target group panels correct each other if they feel someone doesn't take participation duties seriously:

> One of the older persons asks a question about a topic that apparently was already discussed in the previous meeting. The chairperson indicates that the topic will not be discussed further because it was already discussed in-depth. The person coining the question clearly shows she is displeased and claims she was absent the previous meeting. The chairperson corrects her in clear terms: 'but a report about the meeting was made and it's your own responsibility to read those reports'. (Excerpt observation target group panel)

Hence, participation creates obligations and expectations. The strategy of responsibilization can be understood as an attempt to increase symbolic capital, i.e. to become more trustworthy and valued in the medical field by signifying that participation 'duties' are taken seriously.

A third strategy is *pluralization*: i.e. the development of alternative work methods and new fora for target group participation that challenge existing institutional logics. By setting-up alternative fora for participation, some regional networks attempted to prioritize informal work methods, thereby creating more room for the perspective of older persons. The 'regional tables' that were developed in the north of the Netherlands are an example of a small-scale forum in which older persons and professionals exchanged ideas about improving elderly care without a pre-set research agenda or the use of scientific jargon. The goal of these regional tables was to gain more bottom-up input and ideas from older persons and local care and welfare professionals:

> Through older persons I think that different topics are being introduced. They have, for instance, introduced the theme of empathy. What can you do at home for your partner as an informal caregiver, and what do you want yourself, as a person? How do you experience the care you receive? Those were themes older persons introduced and that also encouraged reflection amongst healthcare professionals. (Interview with network coordinator, female)

Rather than following nationally set research themes, the regional tables promoted collaboration between local professionals and older persons and defined improvement themes in a bottom-up way. A consequence of this strategy was that academic research and funding became less the driving force behind participation of older persons. This strategy thus explicitly rejected the subordination of the elderly perspective to the medical field. Although this strategy seemed more useful to enhance the input of older persons, finding enough financial resources to safeguard continuity remained a challenge.

The fourth strategy of *opting out* was used when older persons no longer perceived opportunities to meaningfully engage. Older persons that opted out questioned the dominance of the medical field and the reactive nature of their participation:

> The target group panel was a requirement for the functioning of the projects; it was one of the NPEC requirements. But I felt like 'ok guys, this is not something I want to contribute to'.

Can you explain why you left?

> Well, in general, people (members of target group panels) were fine with commenting on plans (…). But when I was thinking about how to spend my time, I said: 'I don't expect any innovations and the little energy I have left I want to spend on other things (…). The most striking thing is that many people in institutes and public governments don't have a clue how to deal with citizen participation. (Interview with former member of target group panel, male)

When tokenism was expected, opting out seemed the only viable strategy. An important organization for older immigrants for instance turned down requests for involvement from researchers as previous experiences showed that their involvement became a 'check-box' affair (Interview with member of migrant elderly organization, female). The problem of tokenism is well known in literature about community engagement, especially in relation to global health (Arnstein, 1969; Ocloo & Matthews, 2016; Tindana et al., 2007). In the case of the NPEC, one response of older persons experiencing such tokenism was to opt out. While older persons using the strategy of pluralization are attempting to develop alternatives to the predominant rules in the medical field, opting out is more radical and points to a high level of frustration.

These four strategies point to different ways in which members of target group panels have developed responses to the difficulties they experienced in participating. This had some effect: most older persons participating in the panels emphasized that the instrumental view of participation overtime changed for the better. Target group panels were able to gradually change the medical field. This became evident when the funding agency developed specific calls for welfare and started to decline funding to research projects without a connection between health and welfare. Older persons have thus been able to partially adjust the purely medical focus of research that was a consequence of the dominant medical field.

A second effect relates to how older persons were able to convince (part of) the medical community about the importance of their participation. A director of an association for older persons reflects on how the national federation of UMCs eventually published a brochure in which they 'confessed' to the added value of participation:

> The Dutch Federation of University Medical Centres published a brochure (…) about participation of older persons. (In this brochure) they write themselves that they found (this) a nuisance in the beginning: 'and we were annoyed that we had to do this because of NPEC. But we came to love those older persons and we do see the added value now'. So that is a nice brochure because they make a kind of confession, a religious confession: 'it was counterintuitive that we did it, but it proved to be very valuable'. So many of those researchers do say: 'by taking seriously the participation of older persons in my research (….) I have come to see the added value'. (Interview with director of association for older persons, male)

This example shows how older participants have been able to adjust the medical field at least temporarily. Significantly, this 'public confession' of an organization that is an established part of the medical field can also be understood in terms of increased symbolic capital for the community of older participants.

Micro-advantages and disadvantages

The interplay between capital, habitus and field and the strategies employed to deal with tensions in this interplay resulted in the obtainment of certain micro-advantages for particular groups. Especially, the strategies of professionalization and responsibilization turned out to be important in terms of increased social, cultural and symbolic capital. Older persons that were professionalized by training and education were less overwhelmed by medical researchers and the routines in the medical field.

Also, some target group panels were granted specific institutional privileges that increased symbolic capital and enabled further professionalization and responsibilization. One specific target group panel was granted a 'veto-right', which meant that a research proposal would not be submitted for funding if the target group panel decided it was irrelevant. Although this led to criticism from medical researchers, the veto-right increased the symbolic capital (older persons were taken seriously). Consequentially, this also led to an increased sense of responsibility amongst panel members:

> In the beginning, they [the older participants] were distrustful about whether they actually had a veto-right. […] But now they noticed that they were taken very seriously and that had as a consequence that they also took it [the participation] very seriously.

> *How did this show?*

> Well because they had very good discussions and very good arguments about what could work and what wouldn't. So they took their own role [in judging proposals] very seriously. (Interview former network coordinator, female)

Our research also shows that older persons with a large amount of social capital (in terms of a large network to draw on) gained further micro-advantages during the programme. Having a political-managerial network enabled older persons to participate more effectively as they have easy access to relevant organizations (Interview two members of target group panel, both male). Importantly, this also led to an increase in symbolic capital in the medical field as easy access was valued in terms of opportunities for data collection.

Micro-advantages can also work the other way. This can be seen in the way one important member of the national committee, who was a well-respected former politician now taking place in this committee to bring in an elderly perspective, constantly frames herself as ignorant in order to press researchers to change their routines:

> Looking back what surprised me most is the aloofness of a couple of professors (…). Slowly that was getting better. I have emphasized frequently: 'I am a regular girl, I don't get it' (…). They have all studied. I think you need someone from the common folk, like I am. I keep saying that consciously. (Interview elderly representative program committee NPEC, female)

This quote shows that the acquired symbolic capital this respondent gained through her political career in the Dutch Senate allows her to voice a lack of understanding and discipline researchers into changing their routines and jargon.

In sum, having social, cultural and symbolic capital can lead to several micro-advantages, which have the effect that participating older persons are taken more seriously in the medical field. There is also a downside, however: participants lacking the right capital face 'micro-disadvantages' as a consequence of the highly specialized and professional field in which they were operating. For instance, the input of some participants was not taken seriously because they did not use the right jargon or were not able to express their thoughts in a politically sensitive way (Excerpt observation target group panel). This also led to further exclusion processes in which not only researchers, but also participants in target group panels were complicit.

Discussion and conclusion

This paper investigated the following question: How is the inclusion and exclusion of older persons in the NPEC processually shaped through the interplay between individual agency and organizational structures? We have analysed this case of target group participation using the Bourdieusian conceptual framework of capital, habitus and field. We focused on disentangling the relations between institutional context, work routines and the decisions and activities that individual actors employ.

The analysis showed the influence of established fields (medical and policy) on how participation of older persons was shaped in the beginning of the programme, leading to the inclusion of persons with specific forms of social capital and the exclusion of persons lacking this capital. The rules of engagement turned out to be hard to change. Even older persons with much social and cultural capital had difficulties in participating, leading to an increasing recognition that their perspective was used instrumentally. Members of the target group panels developed different strategies to respond to these difficulties. Overall, the voice of community members gradually led to substantive changes in the programme. The strategies of professionalization and responsibilization led to increased social, cultural and symbolic capital for particular groups, along with the obtainment of further micro-advantages. The downside is that participants lacking the right capital face 'micro-disadvantages' as a consequence of the highly specialized and professional field in which they were operating.

In relation to existing participation literature, our study shows similarities and differences. Important similarities can be seen in questions concerning representativeness of the participating group (Trappenburg, 2008; Van de Bovenkamp et al., 2009). The sub-group of literate older persons with a relatively high socio-economic status was not representative in terms of health problems. The question of representativeness becomes more urgent when taking into account the large age differences of older persons involved in the programme, given the differences between the generally more 'resilient' persons of relatively younger age and the more vulnerable and frail groups of very high age that were almost totally precluded from participation. Another similarity can be seen in the strategy of professionalization. The benefits (increased empowerment) and risks (loss of lay perspective) of professionalization are in line with the literature (Callaghan & Wistow, 2006; Van de Bovenkamp et al., 2009). Our analysis shows, however, that the consequences of professionalization cannot be seen as separate from the institutional context and work routines. Additionally, our study shows that other strategies were used by older persons. These strategies led to different micro-advantages and disadvantages (Gengler, 2014). In line with El Enany, Currie, and Lockett (2013), our study demonstrates that not only professionals, but also older persons are complicit in the exclusion of particular user groups.

The Bourdieusian framework offers several analytical advantages. The notions of capital, field and habitus are helpful in exploring the dynamics of inclusion and exclusion, as these processes are neither static nor develop in a social and organizational vacuum. Particularly relevant in this regard is Adler and Kwon's (2002) distinction between 'bridging' and 'bonding' forms of social capital, respectively, fore-grounding external relations or internal ties. As the medical field is well established, it consists largely of 'bonding forms' of social capital focusing on internal ties. Older participants lacking such established disciplines developed 'bridging forms' of social capital to connect to the medical field.

Our analysis of Dutch target group participation in health has wider implications for community engagement in global health. There is a growing recognition that attention for ethics and politics are crucial for the development of 'good' community engagement practices in research. This is evidenced by the increasing number of ethical guidelines for community engagement (Lavery et al., 2010). Yet the impact of these guidelines on biomedical research has been modest (Hasnida et al., 2017; Lavery et al., 2010). Our Bourdieusian framework offers an explanation why ethical guidelines in themselves are insufficient for guaranteeing inclusive engagement. A strongly established institutional field of global health research funding leaves marginalized actors with the need to perform continuous work to have their voices taken seriously. In order to change this, we need more than just ethical guidelines and entrepreneurial individuals. Institutional work needs to be conducted on many levels, including the level of funding (creating new funding structures), research (establishing and maintaining local research infrastructures) and community (new tools and instruments for the embedding of experience-based knowledge can strengthen the capital needed for inclusive engagement).

An important limitation of our framework is that it focuses primarily on talk and action. The concepts allow us to identify what strategies actors develop, what they do and how they talk. Missing from this analysis is a focus on *material* aspects of participation. Especially in the case of frail older persons, such materialities are important as they can give rise to additional exclusion practices (if there is no elevator in the building, participation becomes a practical impossibility).

Our analysis shows that inclusion and exclusion are not static terms but processes that change in the course of a programme. Institutional contexts and disciplinary routines have a major influence on the ways participation is shaped, and it takes time and skill to incrementally change these contexts. We conclude that it is by definition impossible to 'exclude exclusion' at the start of care improvement programmes. It is only in the many pragmatic and mundane choices of 'doing participation' that exclusion and inclusion practices are shaped. Research would therefore benefit from a processual approach in which these mundane practices are followed overtime. Participation is ongoing work and never finished.

Notes

1. It is important to point out that this age range is not the consequence of explicit criteria, but the result of more pragmatic choices by the UMCs to look for 'suitable' participants in their own networks first. Of course, this age range is very broad and has significant consequences. As one reviewer pointed out, people in different age categories are likely to have different priorities, concerns and levels of health. This is something the program committee did not immediately take into account, although recognition of the differences between the more general categories of 'frail' older persons and 'resilient' older persons did become important over the course of the program. While we do not have exact numbers available, we can infer from our interviews and observations that most older persons involved in the target group panels are likely to be between the age of 65 and 80, with some exceptions towards higher and lower ages. There are still large differences and the consequences are reflected upon in the discussion-section.
2. The exact reasons for this are hard to disentangle and also have not been the focus of our research. Tentatively, we can point to three intertwined reasons. First, UMCs primarily searched for pragmatic reasons (such as time pressure) in their own networks, in which ethnic minorities are also likely to be underrepresented. Second, a well-known migrant organization refused to cooperate as they were dissatisfied with the results of previous calls for involvement of minority perspectives in other programs. Third, a wide range of social science research shows that it is difficult to motivate and engage people from minority backgrounds to participate in research activities.
3. The duration of the NPEC was extended to a total of 10 years.

Acknowledgements

We would like to thank Roland Bal and Hester van de Bovenkamp for their valuable feedback which enabled us to significantly improve the paper. In addition, we are grateful to the participants of the Oxford Community Engagement Conference for all the lively discussions and their constructive feedback.

Disclosure statement

The authors report no conflicts of interest.

Funding

This work was supported by the Netherlands Organisation for Health Research and Development [grant number 633300004].

ORCID

Lieke Oldenhof ⓘ http://orcid.org/0000-0001-6188-3933

References

Adler, P. S., & Kwon, S.-W. (2002). Social capital: Prospects for a new concept. The Academy of Management Review, 27(1), 17–40.

Arnstein, S. R. (1969). A ladder of citizen participation. Journal of the American Institute of Planners, 35(4), 216–224.

Bensing, J. (2000). Bridging the gap. The seperate worlds of evidence-based medicine and patient-centered medicine. Patient Education and Counseling, 39(1), 17–25.

Blumer, H. (1954). What is wrong with social theory? *American Sociological Review, 19*(1), 3–10.

Boote, J., Telford, R., & Cooper, C. (2002). Consumer involvement in health research: A review and research agenda. *Health Policy, 61*(2), 213–236.

Bourdieu, P. (1990). *The logic of practice*. Cambridge: Polity.

Bourdieu, P., & Wacquant, L. (2013). Symbolic capital and social classes. *Journal of Classical Sociology, 13*(2), 292–302.

Brown, B., Crawford, P., Nerlich, B., & Koteyko, N. (2008). The habitus of hygiene: Discourses of cleanliness and infection control in nursing work. *Social Science & Medicine, 67*(7), 1047–1055.

Callaghan, G., & Wistow, G. (2006). Publics, patients, citizens, consumers? Power and decision making in primary health care. *Public Administration, 84*(3), 583–601.

De Swaan, A. (1988). *In care of the state*. Cambridge: Polity.

Dean, M. (1999). *Governmentality: Power and rule in modern society*. London: Sage.

Degeling, C., Rock, M., Rogers, W., & Riley, T. (2016). Habitus and responsible dog-ownership: Reconsidering the health promotion implications of 'dog-shaped' holes in people's lives. *Critical Public Health, 26*(2), 191–206.

Dent, M. (2006). Patient choice and medicine in health care: Responsibilization, governance and proto-professionalization. *Public Management Review, 8*(3), 449–462.

Dubbin, L. A., Chang, J. S., & Shim, J. K. (2013). Cultural health capital and the interactional dynamics of patient-centered care. *Social Science & Medicine, 93*, 113–120.

El Enany, N., Currie, G., & Lockett, A. (2013). A paradox in healthcare service development: Professionalization of service users. *Social Science and Medicine, 80*, 24–30.

Gbadegesin, S., & Wendler, D. (2006). Protecting communities in health research from exploitation. *Bioethics, 20*(5), 248–253.

Gengler, A. M. (2014). "I want you to save my kid!" Illness management strategies, access, and inequality at an Elite University Research Hospital. *Journal of Health and Social Behaviour, 55*(3), 342–359.

Hanley, B., Truesdale, A., King, A., Elbourne, D., & Chalmers, I. (2001). Involving consumers in designing, conducting, and interpreting randomised controlled trials: Questionnaire survey. *BMJ, 322*, 519–523.

Hasnida, A., Borst, R. A., Johnson, A. M., Rahmani, N. R., Van Elsland, S. L., & Kok, M. O. (2017). Making health systems research work: Time to shift funding to locally-led research in the South. *The Lancet Global Health, 5*(1), e22–e24.

King, K. F., Kolopack, P., Merritt, M. W., & Lavery, J. V. (2014). Community engagement and the human infrastructure of global health research. *BMC Medical Ethics, 15*(84), 1–6.

Lavery, J. V., Tinadana, P. O., Scott, T. W., Harrington, L. C., Ramsey, J. M., Ytuarte-Nuñez, C., & James, A. A. (2010). Towards a framework for community engagement in global health research. *Trends in Parasitology, 26*(6), 279–283.

Légaré, F., Ratté, S., Gravel, K., & Graham, I. D. (2008). Barriers and facilitators to implementing shared decision-making in clinical practice: Update of a systematic review of health professionals' perceptions. *Patient Education and Counseling, 73*(3), 526–535.

Luxford, K., Safran, D. G., & Delbanco, T. (2011). Promoting patient-centered care: A qualitative study of facilitators and barriers in healthcare organizations with a reputation for improving the patient experience. *International Journal for Quality in Health Care, 23*(5), 510–515.

Montori, V. M., Gafni, A., & Charles, C. (2006). A shared treatment decision-making approach between patients with chronic conditions and their clinicians: The case of diabetes. *Health Expectations, 9*(1), 25–36.

Nutbeam, N. (2008). The evolving concept of health literacy. *Social Science and Medicine, 67*, 2072–2078.

Ocloo, J., & Matthews, R. (2016). From tokenism to empowerment: Progressing patient and public involvement in healthcare improvement. *BMJ Quality & Safety, 25*, 626–632.

Portes, A. (1998). Social capital: Its origins and applications in modern sociology. *Annual Review of Sociology, 24*, 1–24.

Portes, A. (2000). The two meanings of social capital. *Sociological Forum, 15*(1), 1–12.

Ratzan, S. C. (2001). Health literacy: Communication for the public good. *Health Promotion International, 16*, 207–214.

Reay, D. (2004). 'It's all becoming a habitus': Beyond the habitual use of habitus in educational research. *British Journal of Sociology of Education, 25*(4), 431–444.

Rhynas, S. J. (2005). Bourdieu's theory of practice and its potential in nursing research. *Journal of Advanced Nursing, 50*(2), 179–186.

Shim, J. K. (2010). Cultural health capital: A theoretical approach to understanding health care interactions and the dynamics of unequal treatment. *Journal of Health and Social Behavior, 51*(1), 1–15.

Siisiäinen, M. (2003). Two concepts of social capital: Bourdieu vs. Putnam. *International Journal of Contemporary Sociology, 40*(2), 183–204.

Stoebenau, K. (2009). Symbolic capital and health: The case of women's sex work in Antananarivo, Madagascar. *Social Science & Medicine, 68*(11), 2045–2052.

Tindana, P. O., Singh, J. A., Tracy, C. S., Upshur, R. E., Daar, A. S., Singer, P. A., ... Lavery, J. V. (2007). Grand challenges in global health: Community engagement in research in developing countries. *PLoS Medicine, 4*(9), e273.

Trappenburg, M. (2008). *Enough is enough. About healthcare and democracy*. Amsterdam: Amsterdam University Press.

Van de Bovenkamp, H., Trappenburg, M., & Grit, K. (2009). Patient participation in collective decision-making: The Dutch model. *Health Expectations, 13*, 73–85.

Van Hout, M. C. (2011). Assimilation, habitus and drug use among Irish travellers. *Critical Public Health, 21*(2), 203–220.

ZonMw. (2008). Nationaal Programma Ouderenzorg 2008–2011.

Engaging religious leaders to support HIV prevention and care for gays, bisexual men, and other men who have sex with men in coastal Kenya

Evans Gichuru, Bernadette Kombo, Noni Mumba, Salla Sariola, Eduard J. Sanders and Elise M. van der Elst

ABSTRACT

In Kenyan communities, religious leaders are important gatekeepers in matters of health and public morality. In a context that is generally homophobic, religious leaders may aggravate or reduce stigmatization of sexual minorities such as gay and bisexual men, and other men who have sex with men (GBMSM). Literature indicates mixed results in efforts to encourage religious leaders to work effectively and sensitively with issues regarding HIV and sexuality. This paper describes the implementation of an engagement intervention with religious leaders from different denominations, which took place following a homophobic hate attack that was led by local religious leaders, at an HIV research clinic for GBMSM on the Kenyan coast. After the homophobic attack, tailored engagement activities, including a comprehensive four-day online sensitivity training course took place between June 2015 and October 2016 in the Kenyan coast. HIV researchers, together with trained GBMSM activists, organized the series of engagement activities for religious leaders which unfolded iteratively, with each subsequent activity informed by the results of the previous one. Facilitated conversations were used to explore differences and disagreements in relation to questions of scripture, mission, HIV, and human sexuality. As a result, researchers noted that many religious leaders, who initially expressed exceedingly negative attitudes towards GBMSM, started to express far more accepting and supportive views of sexuality, sexual identities, and same-sex relations. This paper describes the changes in religious leaders' discourses relating to GBMSM, and highlights the possibility of using engagement interventions to build trust between research institutes, religious leaders, and GBMSM.

Introduction

In coastal Kenya, HIV-1 incidence in gay and bisexual men and other men who have sex with men (GBMSM) is high. HIV-1 incidence among men who report sex with men exclusively has been estimated at 35.2 (95% CI 23.8–52.1) per 100 person years. These men have a severalfold higher acquisition risk than men who have sex with both men and women, which has been estimated at 5.8 (95% CI 4.2–7.9) per 100 person years, and 1.1 (95% CI: 0.4–2.8) per 100 person years among heterosexual men followed in a HIV at-risk cohort study in coastal Kenya (Sanders et al., 2013). The Kenyan Ministry of Health and the National AIDS Control Council have both called for the involvement and engagement of various vulnerable populations, including GBMSM, in HIV prevention efforts. However, these efforts are obstructed by laws that criminalize consensual homosexual activity (Cohen et al., 2013), often justified by religious deep-rooted prejudice and patterns of stigmatization against GBMSM (Fay et al., 2011; Mbote, Sandfort, Waweru, & Zapfe, 2016; Nordling, 2014).

Kenya is a deeply religious country; more than 80% of the people adhere to a religion. Protestantism (38%) and Catholicism (28%) are the largest denominations. Islam is practiced by about 11% of the total population, and approximately 85% of those living on the Kenyan coast (Kenya National Bureau of Statistics [KNBS], 2009). Religious leaders play a powerful role in shaping many societal issues (Olson, Cadge, & Harrison, 2006), and often present homosexuality as a threat to Africa's religious and cultural norms (Epprecht, 2004; Gaudio, 2009; Lornah, 2013; Thoreson & Cook, 2011). Their rejection of same-sex behavior in African society can negatively impact on health research and HIV intervention work involving GBMSM (Endeshaw et al., 2017; Mbote et al., 2016; Watt, Maman, Jacobson, Laiser, & John, 2009), and indeed in 2010, such attitudes led to the closure of the Kenya Medical Research Institute (KEMRI) HIV research clinic in the coast of Kenya for a week (Samura, 2011).

Reacting to rumors that the HIV research clinic was initiating young men to homosexuality and into same-sex marriages, religious leaders led members of the local community to the attack. GBMSM study participants and staff were the main target. The attack was unexpected but not unprecedented – conflicts between communities and medical researchers have taken place across Africa, suggesting local critique of research and a failure on the part of researchers to engage different community stakeholders (Fairhead, Leach, & Small, 2006; Singh & Mills, 2005; Tappan, 2014). Despite the fact that KEMRI had an extensive community engagement program that strengthened relations with those who participated in research (Marsh, Kamuya, Rowa, Gikonyo, & Molyneux, 2008), and HIV researchers adhered to good participatory practice, such as consulting different community stakeholders from the community advisory board, religious leaders were not sufficiently engaged. Subsequent to the attack, specific community engagement staff was hired to work with religious leaders, to explain the nature of HIV prevention and care research with vulnerable populations, and GBMSM in particular (Kombo et al., 2017).

Engagement activities described in this paper, which we call *engagement intervention*, represent an intensive effort to shape discourses of religious leaders with hopes that religious leaders would change their behaviors, views, and attitudes. Evidence of working with religious leaders in HIV prevention has shown positive results. In an inequitable society like Kenya, religious groups care and support sick and vulnerable people, and thus can enhance HIV prevention efforts (Helman, 2007; Kamau, 2009). Downs et al. showed in a cluster-randomized controlled trial, that educating Tanzanian religious leaders about the prevention benefits of male circumcision led to a higher uptake of circumcision in congregations that had, versus congregations that had not, received the intervention (Downs et al., 2017). Similarly, a cluster-randomized trial conducted by Ezeanoule et al. in Nigeria found that encouraging women at church-run baby showers to be tested for HIV had a positive effect on ART uptake and retention (Ezeanolue et al., 2015). A number of studies have also shown that effectively engaging religious leaders can assist with changing negative public views. Willms et al. showed that collaboration with faith-based organizations encouraged heterosexual couples to use a condom (Willms, Arratia, & Makondesa, 2011), while Cornish with female sex workers in India, and Molyneux et al. with GBMSM in Kenya found that engaging religious leaders contributed to decrease of stigmatization of GBMSM, and supported HIV prevention and care for the most vulnerable and affected populations (Cornish, 2006; Molyneux et al., 2016). For religious leaders, however, it is not easy to denounce discrimination on the basis of sexual orientation, (Agadjanian & Sen, 2007; Miller et al., 2011; Williams, Haire, & Nathan, 2017) and so far, very little has been published on how to engage religious leaders in issues regarding homosexuality in particular. This paper seeks to describe the KEMRI research clinic's engagement intervention and shows that engaging religious leaders can support HIV research and GBMSM access to health care services in Kenya.

Methods

Drawing on the work of Harro (2000) regarding socialization, stigma, and discrimination, we planned a series of specifically tailored engagement sessions with religious leaders, and members from the GBMSM community in Malindi and environs on the Kenyan coast between June 2015 and October 2016. Facilitated conversations were at the center of the activities. Harro's conceptual framework, 'the cycle of socialization', is closely compatible with our prior cross-cultural work with African health care providers on GBMSM stigma (van der Elst, Gichuru et al., 2013; van der Elst, Gichuru et al., 2015; van der Elst, Kombo et al., 2015; van der Elst, Smith et al., 2013), and the literature on GBMSM stigma (Dijkstra et al., 2015). The model built on a set of concepts, deriving from the introductory guide for health care providers working with GBMSM in Africa (Brown, Duby, Scheibe, & Sanders, 2011), and emphasized the overarching context of stigma and discrimination, linked to religious leaders' attitudes, offering possible courses of action to 'choose the direction to change', interrupt the cycle of socialization and potentially dismantle GBMSM oppression.

Between June 2015 and October 2016, a one-day stakeholders' meeting, an open day, a three-day workshop, and six comprehensive four-day online sensitivity training courses were organized with local religious leaders from Malindi and nearby areas in the Kenyan coast. Four members of KEMRI's research team, including two community liaison officers, two HIV behavioral scientists, and six members from coastal GBMSM community-based organizations (CBOs), whose sexual orientation was not shared until the religious leaders had reached a point of being able to receive the information in a non-discriminatory manner, facilitated the engagements. The six GBMSM were trained as facilitators, and had previously assisted with the GBMSM sensitization training for other stakeholders such as health care providers and policy-makers in the Kenyan coast (van der Elst, Gichuru et al., 2015; van der Elst, Kombo et al., 2015).

One hundred thirty-eight out of a total of 141 representatives from six different denominations participated in the engagement activities and included 59 Muslim clerics; 30 Anglican Church pastors; 27 Protestant pastors; 14 Kaya elders (who are considered to be an intrinsic source of ritual power and the origin of cultural identity); four Seventh Day Adventists pastors; and four Catholic priests. All religious leaders were invited on basis of their experiences and visibility in the Malindi community. Three religious leaders refused to participate due to ambiguity regarding the topic.

The engagement activities comprised group work and facilitated conversations, and included an online sensitivity training on GBMSM issues (http://www.marps-africa.org/). This training consisted of four consecutive days of engagement and addressed the following topics: (1) MSM and HIV in sub-Saharan Africa; (2) Stigma; (3) Identity, coming out and disclosure; (4) Anal sex and common sexual practices; (5) HIV and sexually transmitted infections; (6) Mental health, anxiety, depression and substance abuse; (7) HIV prevention measures; and (8) Risk reduction counseling. Twenty-three religious leaders underwent the online training at a time. Modules were designed to be self-completed in 1-2 hours each, and included multiple-choice questions at the end of each module. A score of 71% correct was required to advance to the next module, and upon successful completion of all eight modules, religious leaders were sent a link to download their course certificate. (The learning content of this course is freely available as a web resource and course specifics are documented elsewhere, van der Elst, Smith et al., 2013). Each session was followed by a group discussion, in which religious leaders, and GBMSM and research team members took part.

In each engagement session, facilitators took religious leaders' perspectives (which were generally constituted of prejudicial attitudes, beliefs and stigmatizing behaviors) as a starting point. They used one or two exercises to initiate conversations, deflect tensions and shift focus if needed. Thereafter, they used carefully facilitated conversations to bring religious leaders' conduct, thoughts, and feelings out into the open. These conversations were used to review religious leaders' perspectives of what it means to be human in the society, and what role community and religion play in society at large. Facilitators emphasized the importance of religion in communities, and power that religions and religious leaders wielded. When attitudes of stereotyping, prejudice, and anxiety around homosexuality were uncovered, facilitators applied a carefully crafted approach, and guided the religious leaders through a process of awareness and change within the context of their religious beliefs. For example, facilitators used a commonly shared experience of Kenya's post-election violence in 2007/2008 to deepen religious leaders' understanding of the impacts of prejudices, stigma, and public opinion. Facilitated conversations helped religious leaders to develop an understanding of how stigma leads to discrimination, and how they can be better placed to show empathy and support people who face stigma. After this, facilitators guided religious leaders through a discussion about what they could do to ease stigma and discrimination within their religious communities. Exercises, such as 'turn your habits upside down' (an exercise on the importance of equity, and how religious leaders can support the advancement of equity for all) challenged and helped leaders to critically appraise own attitudes in the context of their leadership in the community.

Facilitators conducted all sessions in Kiswahili, and religious leaders were aware of and consented to the fact that sessions were documented – anonymously – by trained note-takers. Audio recordings were not considered because of participants' concerns about confidentiality. Changes in attitudes, views, and knowledge overtime, were documented in multiple sources of evidence, including reports, minutes, notes, and post-sensitization open-ended evaluation questions. Data were manually coded, translated and triangulated by two researchers (EvdE and BK) using Braun and Clarke's analysis for qualitative data (Braun & Clarke, 2006). An initial coding dictionary was developed through discussions of recurring patterns and themes that emerged from detailed notes and reports generated by the study team (research members, facilitators, and note-takers) immediately after the sessions. This dictionary was periodically updated to reflect nuances and emerging constructs identified during the coding process. An independent (non-coding) research team member (ES) assessed inter-coder reliability to ensure rigor and fidelity to the coding dictionary. Furthermore, data were coded with specific attention to changes in the views of the religious leaders at the start of the engagement as well as later in the process: codes relevant to this paper included themes such as homosexuality is taboo; GBMSM have no place in society; fear and hatred of GBMSM; gap in HIV care and knowledge; shortcoming in engagement with religious leaders; and religious leaders' role in HIV prevention and care. The final analysis presented in this paper emerged after a series of discussions with all team members and included representative quotes that illustrated key findings.

Participants were compensated 1000 Kenyan shillings (approximately $10.00) for their time and transport costs per day. Reimbursement amounts were determined based on previous studies with stakeholder groups, and approved by local representatives and the IRB. Collection of community engagement data is approved by the Ethical Review Board of the Kenya Medical Research Institute and verbal consent is deemed appropriate for anonymous engagement activities.

Findings

Starting point: stigma and insufficient knowledge

At the start of the sessions religious leaders expressed, on the whole, extremely homophobic views. As one Catholic priest, expressing his opinion, said:

> The number of men who have homosexual tendencies are increasing and a danger to our cultural values. (Catholic priest, male)

Several Muslim leaders could not suppress their abhorrence of homosexual men. One said:

> I hate homosexuals and look down at them as lesser beings … (Muslim cleric, male)

These negative views were justified by conservative readings of religious scriptures. As one Catholic priest argued:

> We have all heard of Leviticus, where the Bible straight-up says that homosexual behaviour is an abomination. And yes, it does. It also does say that homosexuals should receive the death penalty. (Catholic priest, male)

Similarly, a Muslim cleric quoted Koranic script Sahih Bukhari 7.72.774,8.82.820:

> Turn such people (GBMSM) out of your houses … (Muslim cleric, male)

Seventh Day Adventists similarly argued that 'gayism should not be endorsed by anyone' and one (displaying his lack of understanding) asked:

> Is there a rehab or seminar that train people to quit [being GBMSM]. (Seventh Day Adventist pastor, male)

A Kaya elder was convinced he could treat homosexuality:

> I normally experience some mystical powers, informed by my dreams. The powers (spirits) can help me treat the individual's [homo] sexuality. (Kaya elder, male)

These negative views towards same-sex sexuality were further justified by religious leaders making references to Kenya's penal code [Sections 162, 163, and 165], which states: 'Carnal knowledge against the order of nature is criminalized'. Religious leaders, however, were divided about whether scripture can be above the rule of law. On the one hand, they generally recognized that Kenya's current constitution also offers protection of civil and human rights which they should also respect. In the sphere of human rights, a Catholic priest cited Luke 10:37, 'the Good Samaritan' and implicated that all humans have a right for their needs to be addressed without concern for race or social status. On the other hand, especially religious leaders who had taken part in the KEMRI research clinic attack were of the opinion that their positions made them responsible to eradicate homosexuality in their communities. This meant that they felt they needed to lead processes of social isolation, or 'pushing out' of the 'sinned' individuals from society.

Negative attitudes were often supported by a lack of sexual education in general and inexperience talking about sexuality in any way. As one clergy from the Anglican Church of Kenya (ACK) shared:

> Since my childhood, I have never heard about coital or non-coital sex ... (ACK clergy, male)

and another leader from the Anglican Church asked:

> How can two men be in love or make love, as sex happens at a place where no reproduction happens ... don't they feel what they do is wrong? (ACK clergy, male)

Although most religious leaders said that their religion had official teaching on human sexuality and that these teachings were described in Holy Scriptures, they strongly felt that religious leaders lacked knowledge about HIV care and prevention. For example, there were myths about the causes of HIV. To paraphrase one of the Kaya leaders, only 'bewitched or cursed' people presented with HIV.

Religious leaders were not clear about their role in supporting HIV care for GBMSM. Yet, they said that there were social expectations that they would have knowledge and skills in these areas. A Protestant pastor expressed his bewilderment at this:

> Many people don't feel comfortable dealing with their sons who are gay and also HIV infected yet they expect us [religious leaders] to advise on a way forward ... but I don't know either ... (Protestant pastor, male)

Responsibility for lack of knowledge of how to combat HIV among GBMSM was partly laid at the door of researchers and those conducting HIV work in the area. Religious leaders mistrusted researchers working with GBMSM and lacked understanding of what the researchers were doing, and why. This was evident in religious leaders' accusations that researchers promote homosexuality. One Muslim leader, who confessed to having been a ringleader in the clinic attack, justified his position thus:

> The lack of community involvement in these initiatives [working with GBMSM] shows that organizations in Africa are funded by Western countries to spread homosexuality. (Muslim leader, male)

Religious leaders identified lack of clear communication and partnership building as major shortcomings of the researchers, and most religious leaders expressed the desire to be further trained on HIV work and stigma reduction toward GBMSM. As a Protestant pastor said:

> Give us information, we have been negligent [and] you kept us ignorant, as community leaders we need to reach many people far and wide ... (Protestant pastor, male)

Changes in religious leaders' discourses relating to GBMSM

Through the engagement processes religious leaders started to generally acknowledge the broader consequences of stigma, particularly in relation to the HIV epidemic. As perspectives changed, most religious leaders started to use alternative scriptures to justify their new perspectives. For example, one female clergy from the Anglican Church said, citing Genesis 1:27:

> We are all created in the image of God, who then knows how God looks like? Why should we judge others with ourselves as the measure? (ACK Reverend, female)

Another clergy cited the story of John (chapter 8 in the Gospel of John in the New Testament of the Christian Bible), saying:

> John 8 tells a story of an adulterous woman who was condemned by the community but Jesus brought her close to help her. This should be our role as religious leaders; to treat everyone with love. (ACK clergy, female)

Another colleague interpreted Peter 2:17, indicating that a change in how religious leaders spoke about homosexuality:

> 'Honor all people. Love the brotherhood. Fear God. Honour the king'. While the Bible disapproves of homosexual acts, it does not condone hatred of homosexuals or homophobia. Instead, we are directed to love everyone. (ACK clergy, female)

These changes were a surprise to religious leaders themselves. A Muslim sheik said:

> I never thought I would sit together with 'mashoga' (gay people) … the training has helped me to build a bridge that I can now sit with them. We have learned those people are amongst us; we are ready to support them and give them counsel. (Muslim sheik, male)

Or, as a 56 year old Kaya elder confessed:

> Since birth I have never had such a training session; 'usilolijua usiku wa giza' (knowledge is power). (Kaya elder, male)

Gaining knowledge about HIV and sexuality *was* particularly empowering for religious leaders and they indicated their recognition that if they changed their attitude towards GBMSM, community members would follow their example. The following quote is of a Seventh Day Adventist pastor:

> Thinking back to our discussions, how we treat HIV, how we treat GBMSM, this [knowledge] is an eye opener … (Seventh Day Adventist pastor, male)

The leaders recognized their authority in mitigating tensions in their respective communities. 'The information we have gotten through the sessions we promise to share it with the wider community and with the interfaith group of Malindi'. They also realized that they have a role to play in facilitating GBMSMs' social acceptance to advance their access to HIV prevention and care. As expressed by a Muslim Clerk:

> At the start of the training we didn't know whether and how we would accept GBMSM in our community … but as we progressed many of us feel that we are now closer to this [GBMSM] community and we have to take the opportunity to set the example, to minister to them as religious leaders. (Muslim clerk, male)

Others indicated that it was an obligation to share their knowledge with their community members. In doing this, one Protestant leader emphasized Hosea 4:6 in the Christian Old Testament, saying:

> 'My people are destroyed for lack of knowledge' … there is need to train religious leaders to equip them with information so that they can reach out to their congregants. (Protestant pastor, male)

Approaches for reducing stigma

The aim of the engagement activities was to support the religious leaders to change their views about GBMSM, and to actively work towards the reduction of stigmatization and increased social acceptance of GBMSM in their respective communities. This required the facilitators to tackle the powerful prejudices and areas of discomfort brought forward by the religious leaders. The research team identified the following key approaches for reducing stigma:

Generate introspection and self-reflection

Religious leaders themselves indicated they had to overcome their own stigma first before being able to guide their congregation and community members. In order to develop self-awareness, the facilitators asked for testimonies of people within the group who had experienced stigma and discrimination. All group members were challenged to listen, interrogate their fears, and show empathy and compassion. This served to provide a safe environment for the GBMSM testimony-givers. Group members were also encouraged to ask questions of the testimony-givers to gain greater clarity on the issues they had not fully understood. GBMSM testimony-givers spoke professionally and openly about their sexuality, and how their sexuality had influenced their social relations. Through subsequent discussions the religious leaders started to understand that they could use their power to influence and persuade community members to follow their lead in alternative ways, i.e. to focus onto developing an understanding of differences between people, lifestyles and the consequences of prejudice, discrimination, and isolation.

Create contact with GBMSM

Having access to GBMSM-members and gay members of KEMRI's research allowed religious leaders to interact with GBMSM to improve mutual understanding. GBMSM life stories and testimonials were used to generate changes in religious leaders' negative attitudes and beliefs toward same-sex sexuality. Leaders explicitly expressed the desire to be regularly in contact with people who have in-depth or at least basic knowledge about various aspects of GBMSM. As one Kaya elder said:

> To be in contact with people who have been in continuous engagement with the GBMSM would help us to reach out to them. (Kaya elder, male)

This was particularly important when male-to-male sexual HIV transmission was discussed.

Provide HIV education

Gaps found in religious leaders' HIV prevention and care knowledge needed to be filled urgently. During online training, brainstorming sessions were used to generate discussion about any issues that came to mind. Small lectures provided conceptual detail, and small group work was used to stimulate participation. Provision of facts, distinguishing myth and gossip from research and truth overcame judgment. Biomedicine was called upon as an expert opinion. This approach, especially when making reference to biological facts, proved a powerful way of reducing stigma. The focus was on improving religious leaders' understanding of why GBMSM are targeted for HIV prevention and care through exposing the leaders to comprehensive knowledge on sexual biology, HIV/AIDS transmission, protection, and treatment. Religious leaders were also provided with knowledge of how to respond as leaders in HIV-related issues. For this, participants brainstormed about ways they could counsel their congregations on HIV. For example, facilitators asked them to devise response strategies for what they would do if a GBMSM parishioner came asking questions about HIV, or if a GBMSM parishioner came saying he had been diagnosed with HIV.

Emphasize responsibility

Sessions placed emphasis on religious leaders' role in supporting HIV prevention and care for GBMSM, setting them at the forefront of the battle against HIV. The importance of religion in communities was acknowledged, and that this provided an opportunity for them to enhance GBMSM's access to HIV prevention and care was emphasized. This happened through discussing religious leaders' counseling role, and the leaders were challenged to acknowledge that it was their responsibility to guide and support GBMSM in a non-judgmental manner.

Require justification

The engagement activities aimed at making religious leaders understand and justify their own opinions and beliefs toward GBMSM within the context of HIV and religion. This was done through group exercises that asked the religious leaders to provide rationale for their prejudices. For instance, religious leaders would prepare a joint sermon on stigma and discrimination using only the messages from the Bible and Quran they would have used before the training. They were then required to role-play and imagine that they were GBMSM members or were living with HIV seated through the sermon. In the same example, religious leaders were asked, guided by questions, to reflect on the tone of their sermon, was it inviting, compassionate and loving or would they feel the sermon was scary and condemning? Would GBMSM be willing to come back to the church or mosque?

Foster researcher relationships

Throughout the sessions, emphasis was placed on calm, respectful attitude and behavior toward each other regardless of differences in opinion. Substantial time was assigned to making the religious leaders feel valued throughout the discussions about the importance of their work. When religious leaders reflected on ethical implications of working with GBMSM members, they mentioned fear to receiving negative treatment from their religious superiors if interacting with this legally defined unaccepted population. With time, however, through continued engagements, religious leaders tended to feel they could freely interact with the GBMSM members of the research team, and express themselves in authentic, relational and self-sharing ways. With encouragement, leaders ascertained that they could sit together, and have a conversation with GBMSM (research) members. This was a situation that before the facilitated engagements they would have resisted. Consensus to collaborate with GBMSM researchers was a concrete step that linked the religious leaders psychologically to the GBMSM members, which can be key to sustaining reduced prejudicial attitudes on a long term.

Two significant positive outcomes materialized after the engagement sessions: a long-term commitment to meetings between religious leaders and the HIV researchers, and the initiation of a 'transformational working group' among the religious leaders themselves to build a strong, united framework that respects individual, community, religious, and cultural diversity, which at the same time focuses on healing GBMSM hurts and challenges mistrust in their communities.

However, social, emotional and spiritual changes are large and complex issues and take time. Although the involvement and commitment of sensitized religious leaders seemed to hold promise for having a powerful impact on ensuring continuous access to HIV care for GBMSM on the coast of Kenya, there were events that we were told about that give us a reason to think that more work is needed. For example, one of the engaged and sensitized religious leaders, who had previously been involved in the homophobic attack at the HIV research clinic, reverted to his 'old' way of talking about GBMSM while addressing a different forum. Another relapse occurred, when one of the positively changed religious leaders was – for some time – ex-communicated by his superiors for having taken part in the engagement activities.

Realizing that lack of endorsement by religious leaders' superiors could limit the effect of community engagements' intention to reduce discrimination against GBMSM, a more holistic approach was then needed. The research team started individual sessions with the religious leaders involved, facilitating personal reflective internal conversation, while the superior, non-sensitized religious leaders, responsible for ex-communication of their colleague, were invited for collective exploration and solution finding. Both the engagements resulted in the same insight deriving from scripture: 'to do unto others as you would do unto yourself', and a concluding variant of the rule: 'to do unto yourself as you would do unto others'.

Discussion

Across the African continent, e.g. in Ethiopia (Endeshaw et al., 2017), Mozambique (Agadjanian & Menjivar, 2011), Nigeria (Ezeanolue et al., 2015), and Tanzania (Watt et al., 2009), responses to the HIV epidemic have involved religious leaders but their support to the HIV prevention and care efforts have been predominantly convergent with religious programs, in form and content. In Kenya, churches and mosques remain conservative in their values about sexuality, and as a result create obstacles to airing social and health problems caused by homophobia, heterosexism, and HIV stigma (Mbote et al., 2016).

Engaging religious leaders from the coast of Kenya resulted in a positive dialog between religious leaders, GBMSM members and HIV researchers. Reflection exercises aided religious leaders to become aware of their own stigmatizing actions and helped transform their habitual use of discriminatory language. Religious leaders also showed that they were able to gradually apply more humanistic, caring discourse, indicating that one can interrupt the cycle of socialization and stand up for change (Harro, 2000). This was possible by supporting religious leaders in their understanding of sexuality and reflection, rather than criticizing or excluding them, or undermining their importance in their respective communities. The reflexive process was instrumental in offering insights to advancing knowledge, and developed a space in which the majority of the group could come to terms with conflicts between religion and recognizing GBMSM existence. Through the engagement sessions the religious leaders became more aware of the activities of the research clinic and felt included and appreciated, rather than left out.

In line with several other studies that have shown that working closely and collaboratively with religious leaders is successful for HIV prevention and care (Duff & Buckingham, 2015; Obong'o, Pichon, Powell, & Williams, 2016; Roman Isler, Eng, Maman, Adimora, & Weiner, 2014; Szaflarski et al., 2013; Taegtmeyer et al., 2013; Williams, Palar, & Derose, 2011; Willms et al., 2011), engagement interventions presented in this paper indicate that when religious leaders reflexively (re)position themselves, changes in views regarding homosexuality can emerge. Our findings, therefore, contribute to existing literature by demonstrating that on-going engagement processes, respectful work, and collaboration in an openly violent environment can generate a more accepting discourse of GBMSM. Given the hostility against same-sex relationships in much of Africa, collaborations with religious leaders are vital, or results can be detrimental as the attack to research clinic suggests.

In Kenya, importance of collaborations with religious leaders is underlined by the fact that the Kenyan state does not recognize the rights of GBMSM. South Africa is the only country in Africa that has decriminalized same-sex relations. Burchardt has shown how rights against sexual and racial discrimination and reasoned secularity have become part of liberal values of individual freedoms and human rights in South Africa (Burchardt, 2015). In Brazil, Muñoz-Laboy and colleagues have shown that historically Brazil's state-defined non-discrimination policies, and closely related national HIV response being channeled through religious organizations, seems to have enhanced GBMSM access to HIV prevention and health care (Munoz-Laboy, Garcia, Moon-Howard, Wilson, & Parker, 2011; Murray, Garcia, Munoz-Laboy, & Parker, 2011). In contrast, in many African countries where decriminalization of homosexuality may be difficult or even impossible in the near future, involvement of, engagement with, and support from religious leaders is essential for creating supportive spaces and access to health care for GBMSM, which, as we have shown, can also enhance community tolerance.

While the results are positive, it is necessary to acknowledge their limitations. First, the sample size was relatively small and not representative of religious leaders elsewhere in the country. Second, the engagement intervention was not planned as a randomized, controlled intervention and thus religious leaders' attitudes were not measured in a structured way. Third and most importantly, the engagement activities cannot claim success in changing every leader in every aspect of their prejudices towards GBMSM. While participants in the process seemed genuinely moved and touched by the process, it is not possible to rule out some social desirability bias in their reported experiences during the engagement. A further study will be required to establish the effect of the engagement intervention on religious leaders' long-term attitudes towards GBMSM, as well as what practical contribution religious leaders may make to support HIV prevention and care for GBMSM.

Conclusion

This study has demonstrated that collaboration between religious leaders, GBMSM members and researchers can achieve notable shifts in knowledge, views and discourses towards GBMSM across a range of religious leaders. The carefully structured participatory processes gave opportunities for religious leaders to interrogate and justify the bases of their perspectives, to reflect on and feel the effects of their attitudes towards GBMSM, and allowed them to engage on an emotional level with GBMSM.

The following recommendations can possibly serve as potentially effective strategies: (1) improve religious leaders' understanding of why GBMSM are targeted for HIV prevention and care; knowledge was particularly empowering for religious leaders as they indicated that if they changed their attitude towards GBMSM, community members would follow their example. (2) Have religious leaders interact with GBMSM to improve mutual understanding and reduce anxiety about interacting with GBMSM. (3) As the religious leaders recognized their authority in mitigating tensions in their respective communities, explain GBMSM research, especially when new initiatives are taken; and (4) Stress religious leaders' central position in the community with the opportunity to enhance GBMSM's access to HIV prevention and care; religious leaders realized that they have a role to play in facilitating GBMSM social acceptance to advance their access to HIV prevention and care. Finally, the engagements with religious leaders in Malindi demonstrated that religious leaders are willing to articulate their judgments differently, given the right support and motivation to do so.

Disclosure statement

No potential conflict of interest was reported by the authors.

Funding

This work was supported by the US Agency for International Development (USAID). Work with key populations in Kilifi, Kenya is funded by the International AIDS Vaccine Initiative. IAVI's work is made possible by generous support from many donors including: The Bill & Melinda Gates Foundation; the Ministry of Foreign Affairs of Denmark; Irish Aid; the Ministry of Finance of Japan; the Ministry of Foreign Affairs of the Netherlands; the Norwegian Agency for Development Cooperation (NORAD); the United Kingdom Department for International Development (DFID), and the United States Agency for International Development (USAID). The full list of IAVI donors is available at www.iavi.org. The KWTRP at the Centre for Geographical Medicine Research-Kilifi is supported by core funding from the Wellcome Trust (grant #077092). The contents are the responsibility of the study authors and do not necessarily reflect the views of USAID, the US government or the Wellcome Trust.

References

Agadjanian, V., & Menjivar, C. (2011). Fighting down the scourge, building up the church: Organisational constraints in religious involvement with HIV/AIDS in Mozambique. *Global Public Health, 6*(Suppl 2), S148–S162.

Agadjanian, V., & Sen, S. (2007). Promises and challenges of faith-based AIDS care and support in Mozambique. *American Journal of Public Health, 97*(2), 362–366.

Braun, V., & Clarke, V. (2006). Using thematic analysis in psychology. *Qualitative Research in Psychology, 3*(2), 77–101.

Brown, B., Duby, Z., Scheibe, A., & Sanders, E. (2011). *An introductory guide for health workers in Africa*. Revised ed. Cape Town: Desmond Tutu HIV Foundation.

Burchardt, M. (2015). *Faith in the time of AIDS: Religion, biopolitics and modernity in South Africa*. Basingstoke: Palgrave Macmillan.

Cohen, M. S., Smith, M. K., Muessig, K. E., Hallett, T. B., Powers, K. A., & Kashuba, A. D. (2013). Antiretroviral treatment of HIV-1 prevents transmission of HIV-1: Where do we go from here? *The Lancet, 382*(9903), 1515–1524.

Cornish, F. (2006). Empowerment to participate: A case study of participation by indian sex workers in HIV prevention: A case study of participation by indian sex workers in HIV prevention. *Journal of Community & Applied Social Psychology, 16*(4), 301–315.

Dijkstra, M., van der Elst, E. M., Micheni, M., Gichuru, E., Musyoki, H., Duby, Z., … Sanders, E. J. (2015). Emerging themes for sensitivity training modules of African healthcare workers attending to men who have sex with men: A systematic review. *International Health, 7*(3), 151–162.

Downs, J. A., Mwakisole, A. H., Chandika, A. B., Lugoba, S., Kassim, R., Laizer, E., … Fitzgerald, D. W. (2017). Educating religious leaders to promote uptake of male circumcision in Tanzania: A cluster randomised trial. *The Lancet, 389*(10074), 1124–1132.

Duff, J. F., & Buckingham, W. W., 3rd (2015). Strengthening of partnerships between the public sector and faith-based groups. *The Lancet, 386*(10005), 1786–1794.

Endeshaw, M., Alemu, S., Andrews, N., Dessie, A., Frey, S., Rawlins, S., … Rao, D. (2017). Involving religious leaders in HIV care and treatment at a university-affiliated hospital in Ethiopia: Application of formative inquiry. *Global Public Health, 12*(4), 416–431.

Epprecht, M. (2004). *Hungochani; The history of a dissident sexuality in Southern Africa; Challenging the stereotypes of African heterosexuality from the precolonial era to the present*. Montreal, QC: McGill-Queen's Universitiy Press.

Ezeanolue, E. E., Obiefune, M. C., Ezeanolue, C. O., Ehiri, J. E., Osuji, A., Ogidi, A. G., … Ogedegbe, G. (2015). Effect of a congregation-based intervention on uptake of HIV testing and linkage to care in pregnant women in Nigeria (Baby Shower): A cluster randomised trial. *The Lancet Global Health, 3*(11), e692–e700.

Fairhead, J., Leach, M., & Small, M. (2006). Where techno-science meets poverty: Medical research and the economy of blood in The Gambia, West Africa. *Social Science and Medicine, 63*(4), 1109–1120.

Fay, H., Baral, S. D., Trapence, G., Motimedi, F., Umar, E., Iipinge, S., … Beyrer, C. (2011). Stigma, health care access, and HIV knowledge among men who have sex with men in Malawi, Namibia, and Botswana. *AIDS and Behavior, 15*(6), 1088–1097.

Gaudio, R. P. (2009). *Allah made us: Sexual outlaws in an Islamic African country*. New York, NY: Wiley.

Harro, B. (2000). The cycle of socialization. In M. Adams, W. Blumenfeld, C. Castaneda, H. Hackman, M. Peters, & X. Zuniga (Eds.), *Readings for diversity and social justice* (2nd ed., pp. 45–52). London: Routledge.

Helman, C. G. (2007). *Health and illness* (5th ed.). Abingdon: Taylor & Francis.

Kamau, N. (2009). *AIDS, sexuality and gender: Experiences of women in Kenyan universities*. Oxford: African Books Collective.

Kenya National Bureau of Statistics (KNBS). (2009). *2009 Census, vol. 2, table 12: Population by religious affiliation*. Retrieved from https://www.opendata.go.ke/1010Religion/2009-Census-Volume-2-Table-12-Population-by-Religi/jrmnkrnf

Kombo, B., Sariola, S., Gichuru, E., Molyneux, S., Sanders, E. J., & van der Elst, E. M. (2017). "Facing our fears": Using facilitated film viewings to engage communities in HIV research involving MSM in Kenya. *Cogent Medicine, 4*(1), 1330728.

Lornah, K. (2013). *SDA pastor preaches against homosexuality*. The Star (Kenya). Retrieved from http://www.the-star.co.ke/news/2013/06/29/sda-pastor-preachesagainst-homosexuality_c794425

Marsh, V., Kamuya, D., Rowa, Y., Gikonyo, C., & Molyneux, S. (2008). Beginning community engagement at a busy biomedical research programme: Experiences from the KEMRI CGMRC-Wellcome Trust Research Programme, Kilifi, Kenya. *Social Science & Medicine, 67*(5), 721–733.

Mbote, D. K., Sandfort, T. G., Waweru, E., & Zapfe, I. A. (2016). Kenyan religious leaders' views on same- sex sexuality and gender nonconformity: Religious freedom versus constitutional rights. *Journal of Sex Research*, 1–12. doi:10.1080/00224499.2016.1255702

Miller, A. N., Kizito, M. N., Mwithia, J. K., Njoroge, L., Ngula, K. W., & Davis, K. (2011). Kenyan pastors' perspectives on communicating about sexual behaviour and HIV. *African Journal of AIDS Research, 10*(3), 271–280.

Molyneux, S., Sariola, S., Allman, D., Dijkstra, M., Gichuru, E., Graham, S. M., … Sanders, E. J. (2016). Public/community engagement in health research with men who have sex with men in sub-Saharan Africa: Challenges and opportunities. *Health Research Policy and Systems, 14*(1), 40.

Munoz-Laboy, M., Garcia, J., Moon-Howard, J., Wilson, P. A., & Parker, R. (2011). Religious responses to HIV and AIDS: Understanding the role of religious cultures and institutions in confronting the epidemic. *Global Public Health, 6*(Suppl 2), S127–S131.

Murray, L. R., Garcia, J., Munoz-Laboy, M., & Parker, R. G. (2011). Strange bedfellows: The Catholic Church and Brazilian National AIDS Program in the response to HIV/AIDS in Brazil. *Social Science & Medicine, 72*(6), 945–952.

Nordling, L. (2014). Homophobia and HIV research: Under siege. *Nature, 509*(7500), 274–275.

Obong'o, C. O., Pichon, L. C., Powell, T. W., & Williams, A. L. (2016). Strengthening partnerships between Black Churches and HIV service providers in the United States. *AIDS Care, 28*(9), 1119–1123.

Olson, L. R., Cadge, W., & Harrison, J. T. (2006). Religion and public opinion about same-sex marriage. *Social Science Quarterly, 87*(2), 340–360.

Roman Isler, M., Eng, E., Maman, S., Adimora, A., & Weiner, B. (2014). Public health and church-based constructions of HIV prevention: Black Baptist perspective. *Health Education Research, 29*(3), 470–484.

Samura, S. (2011, October 25). Africa's last taboo: An investigation into the persecution that gay people face in Africa. [Investigative]. Retrieved from https://www.youtube.com/watch?v=AVp8V1npqyk

Sanders, E. J., Okuku, H. S., Smith, A. D., Mwangome, M., Wahome, E., Fegan, G., … Graham, S. M. (2013). High HIV-1 incidence, correlates of HIV-1 acquisition, and high viral loads following seroconversion among MSM. *AIDS, 27*(3), 437–446.

Singh, J. A., & Mills, E. J. (2005). The abandoned trials of pre-exposure prophylaxis for HIV: What went wrong? *PLoSMed, 2*(9), e234. doi:10.1371/journal.pmed.0020234. PubMed PMID: 16008507; PMCID: PMC1176237

Szaflarski, M., Ritchey, P. N., Jacobson, C. J., Williams, R. H., Baumann Grau, A., Meganathan, K., … Tsevat, J. (2013). Faith-based HIV prevention and counseling programs: Findings from the Cincinnati census of religious congregations. *AIDS and Behavior, 17*(5), 1839–1854.

Taegtmeyer, M., Davies, A., Mwangome, M., van der Elst, E. M., Graham, S. M., Price, M. A., & Sanders, E. J. (2013). Challenges in providing counselling to MSM in highly stigmatized contexts: Results of a qualitative study from Kenya. *PLoS ONE, 8*(6), e64527.

Tappan, J. (2014). Blood work and "rumors" of blood: Nutritional research and insurrection in Buganda, 1935-1970. *International Journal of African Historical Studies, 47*(3), 473.

Thoreson, R., & Cook, S. (2011). Nowhere to turn: Blackmail and extortion of LGBT people in Sub-Saharan Africa. Retrieved from New York: https://www.outrightinternational.org/sites/default/files/484-1.pdf

van der Elst, E. M., Gichuru, E., Muraguri, N., Musyoki, H., Micheni, M., Kombo, B., … Operario, D. (2015). Strengthening healthcare providers' skills to improve HIV services for MSM in Kenya. *AIDS, 29*(Suppl 3), S237–S240.

van der Elst, E. M., Gichuru, E., Omar, A., Kanungi, J., Duby, Z., Midoun, M., … Operario, D. (2013). Experiences of Kenyan healthcare workers providing services to men who have sex with men: Qualitative findings from a sensitivity training programme. *Journal of the International AIDS Society, 16*(Suppl 3), 18741.

van der Elst, E. M., Kombo, B., Gichuru, E., Omar, A., Musyoki, H., Graham, S. M., … Operario, D. (2015). The green shoots of a novel training programme: Progress and identified key actions to providing services to MSM at Kenyan health facilities. *Journal of the International AIDS Society, 18*, 20226.

van der Elst, E. M., Smith, A. D., Gichuru, E., Wahome, E., Musyoki, H., Muraguri, N., … Sanders, E. J. (2013). Men who have sex with men sensitivity training reduces homoprejudice and increases knowledge among Kenyan healthcare providers in coastal Kenya. *Journal of the International AIDS Society, 16*(Suppl 3), 18748.

Watt, M. H., Maman, S., Jacobson, M., Laiser, J., & John, M. (2009). Missed opportunities for religious organizations to support people living with HIV/AIDS: Findings from Tanzania. *AIDS Patient Care and STDs, 23*(5), 389–394.

Williams, K., Haire, B. G., & Nathan, S. (2017). 'They say God punishes people with HIV': Experiences of stigma and discrimination among adults with HIV in Dili, Timor-Leste. *Culture, Health & Sexuality, 19*(10), 1108–1121.

Williams, M. V., Palar, K., & Derose, K. P. (2011). Congregation-based programs to address HIV/AIDS: Elements of successful implementation. *Journal of Urban Health, 88*(3), 517–532.

Willms, D. G., Arratia, M. I., & Makondesa, P. (2011). Can interfaith research partnerships develop new paradigms for condom use and HIV prevention? The implementation of conceptual events in Malawi results in a 'spiritualised condom'. *Sexually Transmitted Infections, 87*(7), 611–615.

Turning the gaze: challenges of involving biomedical researchers in community engagement with research in Patan, Nepal

Siân Aggett ⓘ

ABSTRACT

Global health funding bodies are increasingly promoting and offering specific funding support for public and community engagement activities, in addition to research and programme funding. In the context of this growing commitment to engagement work, we need to find ways to better support contextually appropriate and meaningful exchanges between researchers and community members. I argue that, rather than focusing solely on how to involve communities in engagement with global health research, we should also pay attention to the quality and depth of the involvement of researchers themselves. This is an often overlooked dimension of community engagement in both practice and the literature. In this paper, I present three contextual factors, which created logistical and attitudinal obstacles for researchers' involvement in meaningful engagement in a global health research unit in Nepal. These comprised implicit and explicit messages from funders, institutional and disciplinary hierarchies and educational experiences. Lessons were drawn from an exploration of the successes and failures of two participatory arts projects connected to the research unit in 2015 and 2016. Both projects intended to foster mutual understanding between researchers and members of their research population. As an engagement practitioner and ethnographic researcher, I documented the processes.

Enteric fever is a major public health problem in the Kathmandu valley, Nepal (Karkey et al., 2016). During preliminary conversations about a study designed to trial a water filter intervention, researchers from the Oxford University Clinical Research Programme in Nepal (OUCRU-NP), based at Patan Hospital, experienced resistance to participation in the study from residents within the area. So as to understand community concerns, two participatory arts projects – Sacred Water[1] and Jeewan Jal[2] – were initiated and were led by an artist from Vietnam and myself, respectively. The projects aimed to use conversations and collaborative art-making to generate opportunities for meaningful dialogue between researchers and community members, and to foster appreciation and understanding between the actors involved (Kester, 2004; Phillips, 2011). This aim was achieved with varying degrees of success. I show here, the projects followed the logic (and funder imperatives) of community engagement, but the researchers themselves were difficult to bring into the project activities.

Below, I describe these projects and explore the challenges encountered in involving medical research staff. I found three contextual factors that created obstacles for researcher involvement in engagement activities: implicit and explicit messages from funders that create ambiguity around the value of engagement, institutional and disciplinary hierarchies that influence task prioritisation, and educational experiences that undermine confidence in and the status of creative and dialogic activities. Findings indicate that establishing engagement activities in medical research settings uncritically and without adequate support may fail to create the intended two-way interactions (Research Councils UK [RCUK], 2010).

I argue that funders need to carefully consider what is required of both researchers and engagement practitioners in order to implement community engagement in global health research, and how they might more appropriately encourage and support genuinely dialogical forms of engagement.

Defining public and community engagement

In his recent book on a history of global health, Packard (2016) identified that failure to engage local communities has been a central feature of most global health interventions since the 1930s. Funders of biomedical research, such as the Wellcome Trust and the Bill and Melinda Gates Foundation, are now increasingly offering support for public and community engagement in both locally and internationally funded programmes (Lavery et al., 2010). Still, the definition of engagement can be vague or unclear, and there is a lack of critical conversation regarding the aims and how to achieve them. By definition, 'engagement' differs from the public understanding of science in that it is 'a two-way process, involving interaction and listening, with the goal of generating mutual benefit' (National Coordinating Centre for Public Engagement, n.d.). Community engagement can be traced to development practices brought into global health research in response to a call to see stronger representation and participation of research communities, particularly vulnerable people (MacQueen, Bhan, Frohlich, Holzer, & Sugarman, 2015). Whilst public engagement attempts to engage with a broad and general group of non-specialists, community engagement focuses on a specific group associated with a research programme or project, identified through demographic criteria, geographic area or particular disease (Dunn, 2012; Hamlyn et al., 2015). However, the distinction is not always clear and often the terms are used interchangeably (Aggett, Dunn, & Vincent, 2012), as they are within this article, given that the projects outlined featured outputs (exhibitions) that intended to reach broad audiences, as well as a processes which aimed to foster dialogue and promote understanding between researchers and members of their research community.

It is worth noting that the emphasis within both terms is on engaging those outside of research, rather than engaging researchers. The literature tends to mirror this bias. This is despite concerns being raised that researcher involvement in engagement is not always as committed as hoped. Logistical pressures such as time, resource, reward and recognition, as well as demographic attributes such as age and gender, can influence the inclination of given researchers to engage (Hamlyn et al., 2015). This paper is a provocation to engagement practitioners and researchers to turn the gaze and enter this much-needed conversation.

I use the term 'meaningful engagement' in a considered way. For me, engagement is meaningful when people critically examine their own knowledge and express this without fear, to others who are receptive and responsive to this expression, bearing in mind that there will always be a muddying of the waters in the process of assimilation and interpretation (Falade & Coultas, 2017; Nichter, 2008). This concept of meaningful engagement is principally informed by scholars within international development, and specifically participatory development practice. Whilst engagement might not define itself by the underpinning principles and values purported to ground participatory development (Reason & Bradbury, 2008), parallels can be drawn between participatory development and a wider ethic that community engagement often ascribes to: 'community empowerment', 'raising voice' and promoting 'equitable exchange and mutual understanding'. Therefore, criticism within international development of 'tokenistic' (Bell, 2004), 'manipulative' or 'teleguided' participatory activities (Rahnema, 2010) may also be pertinent to endeavours of engagement in global health. Rahnema (ibid.) indicated that spheres of power around development itself maybe fostering projects with little likelihood of challenging structural forces.

Engagement in global health is situated within wider fields of interest and power, which may or may not permit genuine exchange, community representation or empowerment. Whilst rhetoric promoting engagement in global health may emphasise dialogue, in my experience practice can neglect qualities contingent for dialogue. I believe that in order for engagement to be meaningful, we must pay attention to ensuring that what participants (researchers and community members alike) express is representative rather than tokenism or ventriloquism (Cornwall & Fujita, 2012). In her work on participatory video, Plush (2015) drew attention to the importance of representation alongside recognition of and responses to 'voices raised'. Morrison and Dearden (2013) agree, asserting that in order to avoid tokenism, expressions need to be both 'understandable and deemed valid by health professionals'.

Study context and methods

Patan, also known as Lalitpur, is the second-largest city in the Kathmandu Valley. The Oxford University Clinical Research Unit-Nepal (OURCU-NP) is an infectious disease research unit based at the government-run Patan Hospital. The unit employs approximately 20 staff, all Nepali. They include microbiologists, clinicians, research nurses and community medical assistants (CMAs); the latter do the majority of community-based work, including patient recruitment, treatment delivery and data collection.

The population of Nepal is made up of multiple ethnic identity groups, with differing social and cultural practices. Newar is the most numerous ethnic identity group within the research area, however, increased immigration has brought increased diversification in the demographic of Patan (Gellner & Quigley, 1995). Most senior researchers, although from Kathmandu, were from outside of Patan and belonged to other ethnic/caste identities. This meant that they often had limited knowledge of the customs, relationships and beliefs within their research community compared to others within their research teams, such as the CMAs. With the increase in community-based epidemiological studies since the early 2000s, this has increased importance, and was a principle driver for the projects, which prompted this paper.

Other than some notable exceptions, there is little precedent for public or community engagement with global health research in Nepal.[3] Before the participatory arts projects, Sacred Water and Jeewan Jal, OUCRU-NP's engagement work had been limited to one-on-one interactions to address instrumental needs of research (patient recruitment, consent and data collection), rather than more prolonged interactions aimed at building understanding between researchers and their research community.

The internal drive for a more prolonged and interactive engagement at OUCRU-NP originated from experiences in the design stages of a 2013 community-based study, where Patan community members expressed dissatisfaction with a proposed randomised controlled trial (RCT) of bio-sand water filters. The lead researcher, Dr R, had not predicted a degree of intra-household cohesion, which made the planned randomisation of treatment difficult to justify and to implement. Recognising the need to better understand the research community, Dr R approached the engagement manager at the sister research unit in Vietnam (OUCRU-VN) for support. This led to two projects. The first, Sacred Water, was a participatory arts project conducted over the first half of 2015, led by a Vietnamese artist and funded through a Wellcome Trust International Engagement Award. I led a second participatory arts project, Jeewan Jal, from March to July 2016, which was funded through a Wellcome Trust 'Ethics and Society' award. The former project consisted of a series of arts workshops with female participants from local women's groups. Whereas, Jeewan Jal, worked with an inter-caste and mixed-gender group of 11 young Nepali adults from various academic backgrounds. Both projects explored issues of water and health, and culminated in community exhibitions of artworks. Jeewan Jal also created and performed a community play entitled 'Panika Gunjanharu: Echoes of Water'. Although the participating groups within these two projects differed, both attempted to draw medical research staff into 'engaged' interactions with participants throughout the processes. It is the success or failure of these attempts that are the focus of this paper.

I was invited to support Sacred Water logistically and to include it as a case study in my doctoral research (to explore the potential of participatory arts practice to create spaces for equitable dialogue and knowledge exchange between biomedics and research communities).[4] Jeewan Jal forms a second doctoral case study. I hoped that the projects might deepen researchers' understanding of the complexity of community, including the attitudes, behaviours and knowledge of research subjects (something global health is criticised for overlooking or overly simplifying (Nichter, 2008)).

At the request of the unit director, I conducted a community engagement training session with OUCRU-NP staff, including CMAs, research nurses, the director and other researchers. This took place before either project had begun, and used informal teaching methods eliciting existing interest and understandings of engagement. With attendees' permission, this was sound-recorded, and contributed to the ethnographic data. At the end of the projects, I conducted 11 individual semi-structured interviews (Bryman, 2004) with staff from across levels of seniority. These interviews used thematic prompts developed from the open coding of field-notes (Strauss & Corbin, 1998), which documented informal conversations with staff about the challenges to their involvement in engagement. These included logistical considerations as well as attitudinal and more structural ones. I then transcribed and coded the interviews using NVivo. All data were collected with informants' consent, and has been anonymised as far as possible. Key figures are Dr E, Dr L, Dr R and Dr Y. Other research participants are identified by their professional roles. The research was approved by the University of Sussex's ethics review board.

My research was primarily ethnographic (Brewer, 2000), yet I also drew on participatory and informal learning methods (Chambers, 2002) to explore the relationships, exchanges and knowledge forms circulating within these community engagement processes. Methods drew upon participant observation and field journaling, paying attention to my own relationships, actions and emotions as well as those of others. It involved a lot of 'hanging out' and conversations over cups of tea with research staff in professional spaces of the office or laboratory, or at social events such as public talks and weddings. I was committed to being open, listening and approaching all interactions as a learner.

Findings: challenges involving researchers in engagement activities

Numerous factors generated obstacles for researcher involvement in engagement processes. These fitted within the three overarching contextual factors: implicit and explicit messages from funders that create ambiguity around the value of engagement, institutional and disciplinary hierarchies that influence task prioritisation, and educational experiences that undermine confidence in and the status of creative and dialogic activities.

Implicit and explicit messages from funding institutions

Above, I described the internal impetus for the engagement projects within OUCRU-NP, with the growing recognition that there was a need to better understand the research community. However, the processes were also driven by an external stimulus: efforts to promote engagement from other institutions within the global health network, particularly OUCRU-VN and the Wellcome Trust. The Wellcome Trust – like many other funding bodies – is increasingly encouraging community engagement, using rhetoric around promoting informed and inclusive conversation, dialogue and debate (Wellcome, 2017). Despite this message being implicit in funder behaviour, reporting structures and grant-giving provide clouded, if not contradictory, descriptions and explanations. A representative from the engagement team at Wellcome Trust visited Kathmandu during the Sacred Water project, demonstrating funder commitment. Conversely, there was little formal recognition for research staff involvement in engagement, or other incentive structures such as opportunities for accredited training. This was commented on in the group discussion in advance of the projects:

Discussion Prompt: I would like to do engagement but…?
Programme Director: There is a lack of funds, money, time, authority, approval. I need a trained team.
                                      (OUCRU-NP discussion exercise, January 2015)

The engagement manager in OUCRU-VN, and advisor to Sacred Water and Jeewan Jal, elaborated, stating that 'Funders judge people by the number of publications they have … If it's taking up people's time … away from doing science that can generate a publication, then they won't do it…' There are questions within Wellcome's research grant applications inviting applicants to describe engagement plans; however, the engagement manager confessed, most engagement written into these plans only involves researchers to a cursory degree.

Messages around engagement's aims and values are not necessarily clear in other organisations, nor in the literature (Lavery, 2016). In a time-scarce work environment with little capacity or understanding of engagement, such activities understandably become secondary.

Institutional hierarchies

When I asked whether community engagement was part of medical research work, the answer from all groups interviewed was invariably 'Yes'. However, engagement clearly sat towards the bottom of a hierarchy of valuable work within the research institution. The quantifiable tasks of participant recruitment, data collection and publication were all valued over building understanding within the research community.

It was clear that CMAs felt their work was considered to be less important than the data analysis and publication work of more senior researchers. Dr R spoke of one CMA's feelings after attending an engagement workshop in London: 'He sort of realised that he did important work. That people actually saw his work'. This lack of institutional recognition of community facing work resulted in the people who were tasked with doing it feeling overworked and undervalued. This, in turn, resulted in reluctance to undertake additional engagement-related work. I mused over this with the director, who agreed that engagement was undervalued. As a remedy, he suggested that I try to 'make it look exciting and fun…'

In response, I sought to create engagement activities that could be construed as fun. However, in doing so, I felt a tension. Whilst I argue the value of a playful space in which people and ideas can coincide and interact without conflict, the suggestion was that this should be the principle justification for research staff involvement in these activities. Although it was unintentional, I felt my work belittled, and that the challenges the projects originally hoped to address were at risk of being neglected. In addition, the use of this tack felt discourteous to the CMAs who felt overworked and financially and academically undervalued (not having received permanent contracts after 10 years of service, nor academic recognition in published papers). In the face of their expressed frustration, it felt discourteous to use 'fun' as an inducement.[5] Besides, the members of the research team who might learn most from interacting with participants were more senior staff who encountered the community least in their everyday work. I sensed that 'fun' would not override the perceived importance of their work.

Nonetheless, 'fun' and 'play' were necessary characteristics of the spaces and interactions fostered within Sacred Water and Jeewan Jal. I observed, however, that what I expected to be a positive experience could induce anxiety for researchers; which I will now address.

Accompanying these pronounced hierarchies of professional status, interviews revealed that different researchers held different preferred 'target groups' and associated purposes for engagement. Their preference appeared to be aligned with their professional position. For the unit director, influencing medical practice and policy at a national and district level was the overriding interpretation (and concern):

> Director: So our team should engage up and down the engagement spectrum. On the top would be the Ministry of Health. You know you have to aim big! You have to say 'look, we've done this research and we have published in these journals…' The lowest is going down to the districts.

To Dr B, engagement was very much about clinical relationships and the instrumental needs of research.

> Dr B: The origin of the community engagement concept … is that, say in Africa if you were doing something like the typhoid burden study … in any mass community engagement you would have leaders and consent would be taken from community leaders and their consent would mean, 'Okay you can do it in the community' … We deal with individuals and not with communities…

Dr E was the staff member who gave most time to Jeewan Jal. I asked why she felt engagement was important. Her rationale concerned moral duty:

Dr E: It's giving back to the community. The science, the results, something that you know and then making it aware [sic] in the community in a very different way not in a scientific way but in an easy way so that they could understand it easily.

Those who did not recognise their favoured target groups or justification for engagement within the opportunities offered were less likely to be involved. The director, who indicated an interest in engaging with policy, was verbally supportive, yet neither interacted with nor attended any project events. I suspect that he did not recognise these opportunities as being intended to inform him or other policy influencers, but that rather he understood the projects as community education, with little potential for broader reach. Dr B, who was keen to recruit research subjects, tended towards disseminating promotional information, whereas Dr E felt a moral responsibility to disseminate research knowledge within the community.

It is worth noting that in all instances presented above, the emphasis was on an engagement mode that favoured dissemination and education without incorporating an imperative for researchers to listen and understand, indicating a persisting 'deficit' attitude and disinterest in local knowledge, values and behaviours.

Comfort with creative and dialogic engagement formats

Helguera (2011, p. 45) tabulated two features of engaged encounters: openness or closedness of the format, and directedness of the subject. An open format is one in which participants are creative, in that they have a lot of input into a conversation, such as in a brainstorming activity. A closed format would include a lecture or a speech. I used a mixture of both open and closed formats throughout the project, depending on the project stage, topic and task. Open interactions brought research staff and community participants together without any obvious required outcome other than the very tangible and practical. Conversation was unpredictable, which, permitted some playful, creative and productive exchanges. Open-format encounters included the exhibition launch celebrations and trips to collect prop materials for the play from the hospital. Within Jeewan Jal, an open-format activity included a bus journey to Lele, a village half an hour from Patan and the place of a worshipped water source. Women's group members, young adults and research staff sat together for the journey. Conversation topics were not directed, but the proximity of seating allowed for and encouraged interaction, with serendipitous results. For example, some community participants learned about, and subsequently attained data collection positions at, OUCRU-NP.

At other times an open format was used, but with a more directed subject matter. For example, in Jeewan Jal, research staff were invited to donate water and an accompanying story to our 'museum of water' (a collection of donated water samples with accompanying stories illustrating water and how it features in daily life).[6] They were also invited to offer ideas for reward and penalty cards to be used within our board game, entitled 'Nags and Makars' (see Figure 1) (an equivalent to the game 'Snakes and Ladders', seen played in Patan's communal spaces). Such requests were given in a weekly team meeting and would be followed by an email and face-to-face prompting.

Within both projects, researcher participation was always voluntary. The lead artist would set up the engagement opportunity, invite research staff and hope that they would attend. Frequency and degree of researcher involvement was notably unpredictable. Whilst some team members participated occasionally, garnering longer term or iterative input from any one researcher was difficult. In Sacred Water, invitations to staff to participate in workshops with participants or separate workshops of their own met little positive response. During the Jeewan Jal project, I found that more open formats that invited creative input barely generated any researcher input – only three of the 20 staff donated water to the Museum of Water, and none contributed ideas to our board game. Of the various invitations into engaged interactions, it was the more closed formats, especially if focused on biomedical subject matter, which were the most conducive to researcher input.

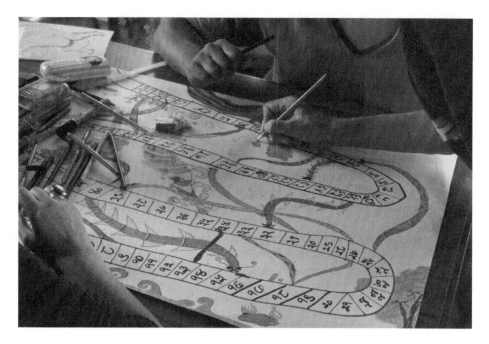

Figure 1. Project participants designing the Nags and Makars board game (based on Snakes and Ladders) (Aggett, 2015a).

This lack of input was perhaps because research staff were intimidated or confused by requests for creative thought. As Dr E reflected,

> The water museum was quite new to me and I was quite impressed with that. Although I couldn't give you the water because I didn't know what I should … [*sic*] But I think that the water museum was a very good idea.

The lack of capacity or the insecurity of research staff preventing them from generating new ideas was explained to me as being a consequence of the Nepali education system, which employs rote learning and hampers the ability to question and think creatively:

> Director: That's the result of rote learning. So the result of rote learning is ah, suffocation. You know? You are stuck in your own rote learning 'five causes of this ten causes of that', when it could be something else.
>
> Siân: And that impacted on people's degree of comfort in doing something as open as I was trying to do?
>
> Director: Exactly. Exactly! And if you encountered resistance in the UK you would encounter more resistance here because of how we have a packaged deal in learning.

This was perhaps compounded by a cultural avoidance of voicing questions, especially amongst women:

> Dr R: In the Nepali culture you don't question especially if you have a male doctor who has worked for 10 years.

Dr R hinted that the challenge I faced might also be due to epistemological differences between the arts and humanities and her epidemiological approach, which tended to look at causal links to proximal and predefined risk factors (Nichter, 2008).

> Dr R: for me everything is facts and everything is in little boxes and then I have got a definite goal … I feel like with social sciences and arts it's very open and you have to be open to get somewhere and I think it is that openness that makes me scared.

Finally, Dr R indicated that there was a conceptual barrier against participating in the arts for those who identify as scientists:

> Dr R: … there is like this age-old thing … with [Standard Leaving Certificates], if you get really good marks and pass in the first division then you study science. If you are average, second division, you study

business commerce and if you fail or are really at the bottom with your marks then you go into arts and social sciences. So here the doctors are like 'Oh, we don't get involved with arts, it's not for us...'

Where moments of creativity were inspired in researchers, it was when there was no obvious pressure for creative performance. Such instances arose in situations where research staff were invited into closed-format interactions where they might expect to educate community members; however, careful facilitation permitted open musing with community participants within these. During such a situation, Dr E (the doctor who had not felt able to contribute water to the museum of water) showed creative ability. She came to talk about her work in the research lab with Jeewan Jal participants who wanted to present the storyline for their play. The group that day was small, and conversation was exploratory and relaxed when Dr E suggested we name a fictional antibiotic which featured in our story 'Wasa-cilin', marrying the standard antibiotic suffix with the Newari word for medicine.

Another process that included notable elements of exploration, creativity and two-way interaction built on a pedagogic structure used in medical school and so was familiar to medical researchers: a directed conversation with discussion points. The structure was open enough to enable conversation within the space, yet closed enough for me to facilitate. Dr R presented her water filter trial design, along with some unexplained questions and challenges she faced in her work. There was little requirement for medical researchers to step out of their area of expertise in this interaction. As part of the process, groups involving both community members and research staff were invited to have a dialogue and to think of explanations for phenomena such as seasonal typhoid patterns or why young men fell ill more than women. Dr R responded respectfully to the group's hypotheses, such as that perhaps migrant males fell ill more readily because they were more likely to drink water outside of the home than women, noting within their responses values, relationships and practices that she had not previously known. In the interaction, she witnessed discriminatory attitudes towards migrant families and their unclean behaviours. This was something she had not learned about in four years of community-based work. She

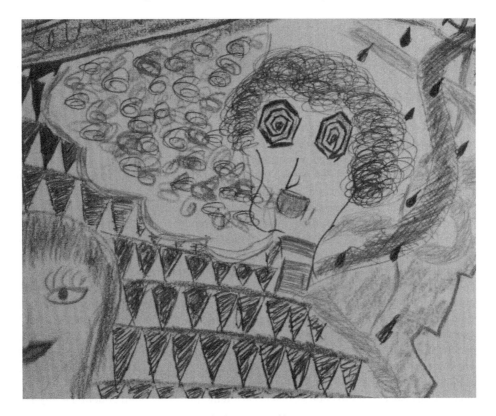

Figure 2. Representation of researcher engagement styles (Aggett, 2015b).

reflected on this, 'That was horrible to hear, to be honest I had never heard that argument before. Even though I went in there and we were distributing water with the water tankers I never saw that'. Later in the session, Dr B arrived. He did not follow the suggested dialogic structure. Rather than discussing research findings and processes, he stood in front of the group and spoke of careers in research in a didactic style, perhaps replicating that in which he had been taught during medical training.

In a separate workshop, after this session, community participants depicted their experience of the discussion in drawing. One group's illustration clearly represented their experiences of the different approaches:

The illustrator explained the picture (see Figure 2), saying:

> The two faces at the corner symbolise the two scientists we interacted with at Patan Hospital. The lady figure at the bottom is Dr R. The white and black background around her represents her study. She shared all her results and outcomes [these are illustrated in white], but she did not have answers to some questions. She was really honest and clear about it [this is illustrated in black]. Dr B on the other hand discussed research methods. As shown in the doodle it was a little confusing for me. (Niraula, 2016)

In sum, closed formats, which replicated educational scenarios with which research staff were familiar (facilitated to retain a degree of openness) appeared to create less anxiety in researchers than open formats (especially when the conversation topic moved outside of their perceived area of expertise). By contrast, facilitating open engagements was easier with community participants, who met more regularly. Therefore, perhaps counter-intuitively, 'semi-closed' formats were most successful in setting up exploratory exchange. Moreover, research staff were better at contributing creatively in informal situations in which they felt unexamined. Didactic roles may have been more comfortable for some of the researchers, but these were less successful in creating two-way exchanges and in conveying information, perhaps because the content was not grounded in participants' existing knowledge or interests but rather in assumptions of these.

Conclusion

Sacred Water and Jeewan Jal were carried out in response to challenges faced by biomedical research-ers in understanding responses to proposed research within Patan. It was hoped that the engagement projects would enable researchers to deepen their understanding of the subjectivities of people within Patan, encouraging more critical thought and perhaps even restructuring how researchers framed research problems and challenges within research design. Neither project, however, succeeded in garnering the degree of involvement from research teams that was required for such self-reflection. Researchers tended to see community resistance as something correctable through education, rather than through engaging in two-way communication (Wynne, 2014).

To some degree, the challenges described in this paper are inherent to any process that brings groups together across power differentials, interests and ways of understanding the world (Helguera, 2011; Rooke, 2013). However, I also suggest that they are particular to engagement in biomedical research contexts, especially in low-income settings where deep hierarchies prevail.

Researchers, perhaps without even realising it, conducted cost–benefit analyses of engagement pro-cesses and – for the most part – found that inducement to engage was lacking. In the projects described, both the funders and the researchers themselves indicated that they wanted engagement, but institu-tional, funder and disciplinary reward systems discouraged involvement. There was no accountability for involvement (or non-involvement), nor were there obvious career-benefitting reasons to be involved. Messaging around funding institutions' policies and priorities, whilst not having complete power over researchers' attitudes towards engagement, can be influential (Palmer & Schibeci, 2012). Involvement in engagement processes was further discouraged by institutional hierarchies, such as the sense that the arts were for people who were less academically gifted than scientists, compounded by an insecurity and avoidance of approaches and formats deemed appropriate for meaningful engagement.

When medical researchers did engage, dialogical interactions were often undermined by a 'deficit' attitude, in which the purpose of engagement was assumed to be about educating people about research findings – accompanied by the assumption that the public would view research more favourably if they were better informed. If, as a thought experiment, we flip this model over, the corresponding argument would be that researcher involvement in engagement processes only requires that the researchers are sufficiently educated to understand the benefits of their involvement. This paper has shown that this is not the case; there are multiple factors that play into researcher resistance to involvement in engagement, and whilst education as to the value of engagement might be one factor, it is not a deciding one.

Efforts at generating engagement were taxing. As a facilitator, I found myself supporting research staff to overcome their discomfort with processes that did not have defined outcomes, needing to curate an unexpected variety of open and closed interactions in order to generate interaction, and having to find subtle mechanisms to engage researchers in dialogue and two-way communications. These were demanding and unanticipated tasks, which were not accounted for in project plans, nor resource and time allocation. These tasks are easily overlooked if we only emphasise the 'community' of 'community engagement with research'.

To conclude, this paper is intended to advance debate in the field of community engagement with global health research by addressing a much-overlooked dimension (the engagement of researchers themselves). Despite the challenges described above, I maintain that the critical approach taken by a strong participatory arts practitioner can allow for in-practice resistance to the expectation of one-way didactic engagement approaches by creating spaces for dialogue between actors who view things from differing vantage points. In order for this to happen, a number of conditions are required. There needs to be a recognition – from funders, researchers and engagement practitioners alike – that the work required of the facilitator to achieve engagement is highly demanding and unpredictable. Funding institutions and other associated academic institutions need to be aware of the role they play in encouraging engagement, and could even consider playing more of a supportive curatorial/ brokering role between practitioners and institutions. Medical researchers need better awareness of the various guiding principles, aims and objectives for engagement, lest activities be destined to slip towards a deficit mode, which most engagement practitioners are keen to leave in the past (Wynne, 2014). Clearer communication and opportunities for experiential and accredited researcher training may support this. Finally, researcher involvement in 'meaningful engagement' over tokenistic engagement efforts must be recognised and rewarded where it takes place.

In order to develop more pointed strategies, we need an equitable, inclusive and critical conversation between funders, research institutions and engagement practitioners about what fairly rewarded and meaningful engagement might look like, and the structural changes required to support these. This ought to include conversations around the possibilities, challenges and responsibilities of involving practitioners from outside of medical research institutions, such as participatory artists/facilitators. Without this, the potentials of independent practitioner-led engagement maybe destined to fail, as they are misunderstood and easily slip to the peripheries of the knowledge project, with it being impossible to encourage anything more than shallow and tokenistic involvement from researchers, thus proliferating rather than contesting existing power structures.

Notes

1. http://www.sacredwaternepal.com
2. https://www.jeewanjal.com/about-the-project
3. Apart from a few exceptions, such as MIRA's (Mother and Infant Research Association) participatory film with rural women's groups (See https://vimeo.com/33243824) and the Nick Simmons Institute's radio docudrama series of health workers' stories (see http://www.nsi.edu.np/?option=com_content&func=details&id=8#.WQr_NIPys1 g).
4. I had a long-standing relationship with OUCRU-VN and OUCRU-NP, having worked with both of these programmes at earlier points in my career.
5. Advice from the senior members of the OUCRU team was that we ought not to pay staff members, as engagement was considered part of their professional responsibility.
6. The Patan Museum of water was inspired by Amy Sharrock's Museum of water (http://www.museumofwater.co.uk).

Acknowledgement

I would like to thank Anna Versfeld: University of Cape Town, Salla Sariola: University of Turku and University of Oxford and Lindsey Reynolds Stellenbosch University and Brown University who provided insight and expertise that greatly assisted the shaping of this research paper, although they may not agree with all of the interpretations/conclusions of this paper.

Disclosure statement

No potential conflict of interest was reported by the author.

Funding

This research was conducted as part of my doctoral research funded under a Wellcome Trust Ethics and Society Award (Wellcome Grant Number-102021/Z/13/Z) This article was based on in-depth interviews and ethnographic journaling. Due to ethical concerns, supporting data cannot be made openly available.

ORCID

Siân Aggett http://orcid.org/0000-0001-8271-2949

References

Aggett, S. (2015a). Figure 1 [Jeewan Jal Workshop Photograph].

Aggett, S. (2015b). Figure 2 [Jeewan Jal Workshop Photograph].

Aggett, S., Dunn, A., & Vincent, R. (2012). *Engaging with impact: How do we know if we have made a difference?*. London: Wellcome Trust.

Bell, S. (2004). Does 'participatory development' encourage processes of empowerment? *Centre for Developing Areas Research, Research Paper*, 41.

Brewer, J. D. (2000). *Ethnography*. Buckingham and Philadelphia: Open University Press.

Bryman, A. (2004). *Social research methods* (2nd ed.). Oxford: Oxford University Press.

Chambers, R. (2002). *Participatory Workshops: A sourcebook of 21 sets of ideas and activities*. London: Earthscan.

Cornwall, A., & Fujita, M. (2012). Ventriloquising 'the Poor'? Of voices, choices and the politics of 'participatory' knowledge production. *Third World Quarterly, 33*(9), 1751–1765.

Dunn, A. (2012). *Community engagement under the microscope*. (Workshop Report). London: Wellcome Trust.

Falade, B. A., & Coultas, C. J. (2017). Scientific and non-scientific information in the uptake of health information: The case of Ebola. *South African Journal of Science, 113*(7/8), 1–8.

Gellner, D., & Quigley, D. (1995). *Contested hierarchies: A collaborative ethnography of caste among the Newars of the Kathmandu Valley, Nepal*. Oxford: Clarendon Press.

Hamlyn, B., Shanahan, M., Lewis, H., O'Donoghue, E., Hanson, T., & Burchell, K. (2015). *Factors affecting public engagement by researchers: A study on behalf of a consortium of UK public research funders*. London: Wellcome Trust.

Helguera, P. (2011). *Education for socially engaged Arts: A materials and techniques handbook*. New York, NY: Jorge Pinto Books.

Karkey, A., Jombart, T., Walker, A., Thompson, C. N., Torres, A., Dongol, S., & Baker, S. (2016). The ecological dynamics of faecal contamination and Salmonella typhi and Salmonella paratyphi A in municipal Kathmandu drinking water. *PLOS Neglected Tropical Diseases, 10*(1) 1–8.

Kester, G. (2004). *Conversation pieces: Community + communication in modern art*. Los Angeles, CA: University of California Press.

Lavery, J. (2016, April). *A working model of community engagement*. Paper presented at the Bill & Melinda Gates Foundation Malaria.

Lavery, J., Tindana, P., Scott, T., Harrington, L., Ramsey, J., Ytuarte-Nuñez, C., & James, A. (2010). Towards a framework for community engagement in global health research. *Trends in Parasitology, 6*, 279–283.

MacQueen, K., Bhan, A., Frohlich, J., Holzer, J., & Sugarman, J. (2015). Evaluating community engagement in global health research: The need for metrics. *BMC Medical Ethics, 16*(1), 44.

Morrison, C., & Dearden, A. (2013). Beyond tokenistic participation: Using representational artefacts to enable meaningful public participation in health service design. *Health Policy, 112*(3), 179–186.

National Coordinating Centre for Public Engagement. (n.d.). Retrieved from https://www.publicengagement.ac.uk/explore-it/what-public-engagement

Nichter, M. (2008). *Global health: Why cultural perceptions, social representations, and biopolitics matter*. Tuscon, AZ: University of Arizona Press.

Niraula, D. (2016). Conversation pieces doodles [drawing]. Retrieved from https://www.jeewanjal.com/single-post/2016/04/22/Conversation-PiecesDoodles

Packard, R. (2016). *A history of global health: Interventions into the lives of other peoples.* Baltimore, MD: John Hopkins University Press.

Palmer, S., & Schibeci, R. (2012). What conceptions of science communication are espoused by science research funding bodies? *Public Understanding of Science, 23*(5), 511–527.

Phillips, L. (2011). *The promise of dialogue. The dialogic turn in the production and communication of knowledge.* Amsterdam: John Benjamins Publishing Company.

Plush, T. (2015). Participatory video and citizen voice – We've raised their voices: Is anyone listening? *Glocal Times, 22*(23), 1–16.

Rahnema, M. (2010). Participation. In W. Sachs (Ed.), *The development dictionary: A Guide to knowledge as power* (2nd ed.). London: Zed Books.

Reason, P., & Bradbury, H. (Eds.). (2008). *Handbook of action research: Participative inquiry and practice* (2nd ed.). London: Sage.

Research Councils UK. (2010). *Concordat for engaging the public with research.* Swindon: RCUK RCUK. Retrieved from http://www.rcuk.ac.uk/per/Pages/Concordat.aspx

Rooke, A. (2013). *Curating community The relational and agonistic value of participatory arts in superdiverse localities.* Discussion Paper. Arts and Humanities Research Council.

Strauss, A., & Corbin, J. (1998). *Basics of qualitative research techniques and procedures for developing grounded theory* (2nd ed.). London: Sage.

Wellcome. (2017) Provision for public engagement within research grants. Retrieved from https://wellcome.ac.uk/funding/public-engagement-funding-within-research-grants

Wynne, B. (2014). Further disorientation in the hall of mirrors. *Public Understanding of Science, 23*(1), 60–70.

Speaking for others: ethical and political dilemmas of research in global health

Abhilasha Karkey (iD) and Judith Green (iD)

Researchers inevitably present partial views of the worlds they study. Decisions about what to include and exclude are shaped by disciplinary foci, current debates and imagined audiences. No research is ever complete: all findings reveal new areas of ignorance and fresh questions for enquiry. But if research reports can never be comprehensive, they should be credible, with inferences warranted on the data presented. When the field of research is one's actual or potential collaborators – reflective agents who are also insightful analysts of the same worlds – debate around inference and credibility can become fraught. When those collaborations are between those with differential access to power, this debate becomes entangled with the politics and ethics of global, disciplinary, and other inequities.

The first author of this chapter was in the uncomfortable position of being part of the field reported on in a recent paper (Aggett, 2018). This paper argued that there were limitations in including medical researchers as part of the processes of community engagement in a setting in Nepal. As an 'insider' in the field, Karkey had a number of concerns about the interpretations offered in the paper, specifically around: the extent to which the community were 'resistant', as claimed; the claim that community medical assistants were not recognized in published papers and the claim that senior staff had little contact with the local community. Karkey also felt the paper was unnecessarily judgemental about the local limitations of participatory processes, countering that progress is inevitably slow, with trust built incrementally over many years, and that local successes in vaccination programmes attest to good relationships with local communities. These different interpretations of the same field generate questions around how far any 'outsider', with limited language fluency, even one who has worked and studied there over time, can be a reliable informant on such issues as the intricacies of caste and ethnicity, or whether local practitioners understand community beliefs. How can outsiders comment on issues such as lack of permanent contracts, for instance, with little understanding of local economies or working practices?

Of course such questions are commonplace critiques of traditional ethnography, and its limited ability to speak for an 'other' who can be only partially understood. All ethnography, perhaps, entails betrayal (Fine, 1993). What is gained analytically by the outsider status should offset these limitations: fresh insights, informed by theory, and a critical and holistic grasp of what is going on. But as research subjects, rendered as local, most of us, when our life's work is subject to critique, would struggle to avoid feelings of betrayal and misrepresentation. Anthropologists are increasingly in positions where their 'subjects' are also colleagues. David Mosse (2006), for instance, has written about objections some of his colleagues made at his draft account of an ethnography of international aid, and the long processes of critique he was subjected to (including being reported to his professional association for breach of ethical guidelines) before the report could be published. His ethnography had been read as evaluation, and as judgement, and some questioned both his credibility and his ethical position. As he notes, questions of veracity are difficult to defend in such ethnographies: both the subject and the author 'were there'. For Mosse, one implication is that ethnography continues after the fieldwork: the processes of critique and defence are part of the ongoing task of exploring the field. As he puts it: 'Anthropologists have the power to represent; and their informants have different capacities to object' (Mosse, 2006, p. 951)

However, the power of informants to object is not, of course, evenly distributed. Mosse was 'studying up', and could perhaps take the moral high ground of speaking truth to powerful elites who had at their disposal a range of strategies to curtail narratives that were unwelcome. Less well-resourced informants may be limited to shunning future collaboration with the ethnographer (Scheper-Hughes, 2000), deflecting enquiry, or using deception and other 'weapons of the weak' (Scott, 1985). Elites have more power to resist scrutiny in the first place, to restrict the narratives available about them, and to reframe those that do get into the public domain. Yet identifying who has power is not straightforward: it can be held in some domains and not others, and is not necessarily unidirectional. In global partnerships, southern partners (whether the researcher or the researched) face greater challenges in objecting to depictions of their worlds. They have less access to fora such as international academic journals or policy agenda, and fewer opportunities to access research funding to create their own narratives (Bezuidenhout, Kelly, Leonelli, & Rappert, 2017). But relative powerlessness is not homogenous: the interests of civil servants, biomedical doctors, other health professionals, their clients, and other communities are unlikely to be neatly aligned. In revealing such divisions, or speaking for the most marginalized, researchers from the global north risk alienating other constituencies, with consequences which can be difficult to predict. As Cooke and Kothari (2001) argue, participatory research is a risky endeavour in this regard: potentially obscuring rather than revealing both legitimate local democratic processes and structures of power. However, the researchers from northern partners are not necessarily in the most powerful position: their own employment may be precarious and dependent on relations of patronage. Fieldwork is often done early in a career, when the continued goodwill of a range of collaborators and mentors is essential. As social scientists, they may be subordinates within medicalized research and policy hierarchies.

Reflexive engagement with ethical guidance is a necessary, but hardly sufficient, requirement for navigating these complex and cross-cutting power relationships in global health research. To volunteer to be studied is to place oneself in a potentially vulnerable position. Ethical guidance, particularly requirements for informed consent, is designed to protect the research subject, but for most qualitative research it is of course impossible to fully inform participants of what is likely to happen to the data they generate before the analysis is done, or to predict what will happen to future research reports when they are out in the world. And even if it were, it is perhaps impossible to image how it feels to read another's account of your world until you do. Assurances of confidentiality may mean little: the damage is not to the esteem with which you are held in the world, but to self-image. The whole notion of 'informed consent' has been critiqued in ethnography (Bell, 2014) as an inappropriate creep from biomedicine. This is not to say that ethnographers have no ethical obligations and that they should not ordinarily seek to secure meaningful, ongoing consent to be in the field – only that there are real limitations in our abilities to realistically outline the 'risks and benefits' of taking part in an ethnographic study.

So what should critical public health scholars do? Given that all research reports are partial, the risks of generating criticisms of betrayal, suggestions of 'parachute' global health journalism, and misrepresentation are real, and all too common. We should, therefore, first ensure that our practices acknowledge their own limitations. In pragmatic terms, there are a number of strategies that can be useful. Probably the most important is sharing drafts with a range of others, including key informants, before publication. This practice can not only offset the dangers of getting matters of fact wrong, but can potentially generate fruitful lines of analytical enquiry, through accounting for disparate interpretations. Could collaborating on writing with the hosts and including disparate views have enriched the analysis? Journal reviewers and editors also have a role in considering some difficult questions during the review process: is the interpretation credible and robust? Should there have been other co-authors, if the paper appears to have been emerged from a collaborative research endeavour? This is perhaps particularly pertinent when the report is by a single author from the global north, and the setting in a low/middle income country. There are also implications for academic publishing. Moves to digital publication might enlarge the spaces for more fluid publications, with rights of reply and debate, rather than static journal papers which suggest the final word.

ORCID

Abhilasha Karkey ⓘ http://orcid.org/0000-0002-5179-650X
Judith Green ⓘ http://orcid.org/0000-0002-2315-5326

References

Aggett, S. (2018). Turning the gaze: Challenges of involving biomedical researchers in community engagement with research in Patan, Nepal. *Critical Public Health, 28*(3), 306–317.

Bell, K. (2014). Resisting commensurability: Against informed consent as an anthropological virtue. *American Anthropologist, 116*(3), 511–522.

Bezuidenhout, L., Kelly, A. H., Leonelli, S., & Rappert, B. (2017). '$100 is not much to you': Open science and neglected accessibilities for scientific research in Africa. *Critical Public Health, 27*(1), 39–49.

Cooke, B., & Kothari, U. (Eds.). (2001). *Participation: The new tyranny?* London: Zed books.

Fine, G. A. (1993). Ten lies of ethnography: Moral dilemmas of field research. *Journal of Contemporary Ethnography, 22*(3), 267–294.

Mosse, D. (2006). Anti-social anthropology? Objectivity, objection, and the ethnography of public policy and professional communities. *Journal of the Royal Anthropological Institute, 12*(4), 935–956.

Scheper-Hughes, N. (2000). Ire in Ireland. *Ethnography, 1*(1), 117–140.

Scott, J. C. (1985). *Weapons of the weak: Everyday forms of peasant resistance*. New Haven: Yale University Press.

Who is answerable to whom? Exploring the complex relationship between researchers, community and Community Advisory Board (CAB) members in two research studies in Zambia

Musonda Simwinga, John Porter and Virginia Bond

ABSTRACT

This paper explores the accountability relationships that arise between researchers, the community and community representative structures known as Community Advisory Boards (CABs). It draws on ethnographic and case study research that documented the history, recruitment, composition and representativeness of two CABs and their relationships with researchers and communities, carried out in two studies in Zambia between 2010 and 2014. The findings revealed contradictions, nuances and imbalances in actual community participation and representation. In both studies, the general population was not given the opportunity to participate in the election of their CAB representatives, and the elected CAB members themselves were initially told to have little or no direct contact with research participants whom they were supposed to represent (unless researchers dictated otherwise). Owing to the researchers' monopoly of scientific knowledge, literacy and financial resources, power relations were imbalanced. Further, researchers were quick to ask for and formalise community commitment through the CABs whilst reticent about their own accountability to the community. Yet despite these imbalances and CABs lacking formal authority over researchers, CABs did have subtle powers arising from their wider influence in the community, which they could tap into to either support or resist research. To achieve a more balanced and open accountability between research stakeholders, more genuine participatory processes need to be built and sustained.

Introduction

Community-based research in Africa is often initiated by researchers who have considerable skills, knowledge and financial resources. Yet to conduct research that is successful and that adheres to international guidelines, active participation of local residents is necessary (Becker, Israel, Gustat, Reyes, & Allen III, 2013; Tindana et al., 2007). In fact, participation of local residents in all stages of the research process is encouraged (Dickert & Sugarman, 2005; Minkler, Blackwell, Thompson, & Tamir, 2003; Woolf, Zimmerman, Haley, & Krist, 2016). 'Community engagement' has thus become a standard practice in research programmes in sub-Saharan Africa. It has several desired ends, including securing permission to enter community settings, soliciting input into studies and ensuring ongoing dialogue. In bioethical discourse, community engagement is considered as an inclusive and empowering process. By developing meaningful partnerships with the people who are part of and familiar with the broader social, political and economic environments within which research is being conducted, community engagement is intended to ensure that research is relevant, protects and respects communities and participants, minimises the possibility of exploitation by researchers, and has a high chance of positively impacting communities (Israel, Schulz, Parker, & Becker, 1998; MacQueen, Bhan, Frohlich, Holzer, & Sugarman, 2015; Macqueen, Kerry, Alleman, Mcclain Burke, & Mack, 2006).

Although community engagement can take on many forms (several of which are explored in this special issue), one of the most common ones is the community advisory board (CAB). CABs are organised groups of individuals, usually volunteers, appointed or elected by 'the community' to represent its interests by providing input in the research process (Wakefield, 2005). CABs may be established to serve one study or many (Quinn, 2004). They are set up to perform a variety of functions. Aside from government and Institutional Review Boards/ Ethics Committees, CABs are frequently among the first groups that facilitate the entry of research studies into communities. With medical research often embedded in colonialism, residents may not trust the researchers in the absence of recognisable community representatives, and therefore CABs are considered to play an important role in building trust. CABs are also intended to provide organisation and leadership to the collaboration between researchers and communities (Newman, Andrews, Magwood, Jenkins, Cox, & Williamson, 2011). Perhaps most importantly CABs are considered as a meaningful and effective way of countering the potential of exploitation in international research (Pratt et al., 2015).

The ability of CABs to represent community interests and to reduce exploitation depends to a large extent on the accountability mechanisms between researchers, CABs and the people they represent. Accountability can be understood as a 'referee of the dynamics in two-way relationships' (George, 2003) often between entities, organisations or individuals who may not have equal power or influence. Accountability can also be understood in terms of answerability, meaning that (research) organisations are obliged to answer to partners, provide them with information and justify their actions (Brinkerhoff, 2004). A small number of studies have suggested that, in practice, CABs often have very limited powers and ability to demand and enforce accountability. CABs have been described as 'paper councils' or 'window dressers' (Cox, Rouff, Svendsen, Markowitz, & Abrams, 1998; Strauss et al., 2001), lacking the power to influence the research agenda and to reduce the potential for exploitation (Pratt et al., 2015; Slevin, Ukpong, & Heise, 2008). CABs can in this regard be viewed as appendages to research with the specific interest of enrolling the world's most poor and vulnerable into clinical trials (Nguyen, 2015; Petryna, 2009; Rottenburg, 2009). Yet we still have very few sustained accounts of how CABs perceive their roles, how they balance their allegiances between researchers and community members and how they strive to demand and enforce accountability.

To increase our understanding of the accountability relationships between researchers, CABs and study communities, this paper draws on ethnographic and case study research with two CABs in the two medical research studies in Zambia conducted between 2010 and 2014. At the heart of this paper lies a concern with who, in practice, is answerable to whom. The findings revealed inherent power imbalances in the three layers of accountability relationships; between CABs and the community, between CABs and researchers and between researchers and CABs/community. The monopoly of scientific knowledge, literacy and financial resources of the researcher accentuated this imbalance. However, CABs had subtle powers arising from their wider influence in the community that partially offset this imbalance. To further tap into this broad-based influence and to make researchers more genuinely accountable, we argue for more participatory processes.

Study setting and methods

This paper is based on PhD research conducted by the first author to explore the role and function of CABs. The research was nested within two ongoing studies in Zambia which we refer to, respectively, as (1) the Human Immunodeficiency Virus (HIV) study and (2) the Tuberculosis (TB) study. They were conducted in two high-density urban areas in Lusaka: Maliko and Kapata (pseudonyms), respectively. The HIV study was a multi-site observational cohort study aimed at understanding trends over time of sexual HIV transmission risk behaviour in HIV positive individuals under treatment. The TB study was a randomised placebo-controlled double-blind study comparing two shortened regimes for TB treatment. Recruitment of study participants was conducted within two health facilities which serviced the two respective geographical communities. Ethical approval was obtained from the University of Zambia (UNZA) Biomedical Ethics Committee and the Ethics Committee of the London School of Hygiene and Tropical Medicine. Written informed consent was obtained from all participants.

An ethnographic study design and case study analytic approach was used as this approach is ideally suited for exploring social relationships through interactions with research participants (Liamputtong & Ezzy, 2005; Merriam, 2009). The first author and a research assistant spent time in the field attending CAB and sensitisation meetings and observing CAB members and researchers interact in different forums.

The case study approach (Green & Thorogood, 2009) helps to illuminate cases in great depth and detail (Murray & Beglar, 2009) using different data collection methods. Accordingly, a mix of methods was used to triangulate the findings from the CABs in the two studies. In-depth interviews ($n = 25$) with CAB members and researchers were conducted, and, to assess individuals' experiences, key informant interviews ($n =$ nine) were done with purposely selected residents who had knowledge of the community (opinion leaders) (Richards, 2009). Secondly, focus group discussions ($n =$ nine) with members of the community were used to understand collective narratives. For a year and half, observations of research activities ($n = 33$) were conducted to enable a deeper understanding of behaviour and interactions (Silverman, 2011). Finally, participatory research appraisal techniques were employed to gather background information for both communities. These included asking residents ($n =$ eight) who had knowledge of and who had lived in the community for at least 10 years, to draw social maps and to construct historical timelines of the two communities. Selection of information rich residents for in-depth interviews and participatory appraisal research activities was carried out with the help of a local Community-Based Organisation, the Neighbourhood Health Committee which works with health facility management to identify and mitigate health challenges in communities. A Neighbourhood Health Committee was present in both communities. In addition, document analysis ($n = 35$) was conducted to gain insight into unobservable interactions. This included documents of: CAB meeting minutes, community meetings and sensitisation reports, CAB guidelines or constitution, correspondence between researchers and the CABs, study instruments and any form of records that were kept by the studies and CABs on CAB activities. All focus group discussions, participatory research appraisal and document analysis were conducted by the first author with some observations and interviews carried out by the research assistant. Interview guides and observation checklists were developed and piloted.

All interviews were recorded, while observations and data from participatory research appraisal activities were written up as field notes using a guide which divided the observations into two broad categories; field activities and meetings and or forums in which researchers interacted with the CABs and the community. Interviews conducted in the local language (Nyanja and Bemba) were first transcribed and then translated into English and were then imported into NVivo. A code book (thematic framework) was developed by the first author, with assistance from the supervisors and research assistant, consisting of both preconceived themes from the study's conceptual framework and themes which emerged from the field data. This was followed by coding of the data by the first author. Data were then charted into different matrices and tables bearing themes or variables for interpretation of the data across participants, themes and communities.

Findings

Themes identified through thematic analysis included the formation and composition of the CAB, the development of the CAB selection criteria, and the nature of interactions and power relations between researchers and the CABs. Other related themes included representation and legitimacy. These themes were presented and discussed in relation to accountability, leading to the identification of three layers of accountability relationships: the relationship between CABs and the community, between CABs and researchers and the relationship between researchers and the community.

CAB formation, composition and selection of members

According to the researchers, CABs were formed to enhance community engagement through the provision of feedback, 'community voice' and advice regarding sensitisation, recruitment and retention activities. The CAB for the HIV study was formed before the start of the study, while the CAB for the TB study was created after the study had already commenced. Prior to the establishment of the CAB, the Neighbourhood Health Committee played the CAB's role. The timing of the creation of the CAB was important as it determined how much influence the community had in the design and subsequent processes of the study. The CAB for the HIV study was composed of five members – three men and two women – while the CAB for the TB study was composed of 13 members, five men and eight women. The 13 members of the TB study CAB represented 12 Community-Based Organisations and other inter-est groups. Some members belonged to more than one Community-Based Organisation and several were also members of respective Neighbourhood Health Committees. All the HIV study CAB members completed senior secondary school and four attained college education and were formerly employed. In comparison, only four of the thirteen TB study CAB members had completed senior education, and only three had attained a college education. The composition of the CAB was important because it reflected a broad representation of community interests and geographical spread.

The CAB members in both studies were selected using criteria determined by researchers, rather than community residents themselves. Using different criteria and guidelines, CAB members were selected with the help of the Neighbourhood Health Committees and health facility management. Some Community-Based Organisations were asked to nominate a representative using the set criteria. Of these, literacy and education were considered the most important. CAB members were required to be able to read and write, at least in their local language but preferably in English too. In the CAB of the HIV study, most members were proficient in both; but in the case of the TB CAB, some of the members struggled to read and write in English and CAB meetings were conducted in a mix of local languages and English. Observations of CAB meetings showed that comprehension was still a challenge for some CAB members. Yet the selection of literate individuals was meant to assure some level of research com-prehension and by extension, increase CAB answerability to the community.

Age requirements were not explicitly stated in the guidelines/criteria. Nonetheless, all CAB mem-bers were either middle aged or older, ranging between 35 and 65 years old. Members of both CABs expressed that they considered young persons as too immature to serve on the CABs and that they may not have sufficient time as they were supposed to be in school. The reality, however, was that young people often held volunteer roles at the health facilities. Both CABs experienced high attrition in their early stages of development because some members had expected higher compensations and attendant benefits than they were offered.

Place of residence was also viewed as an important selection criterion and people residing within the community were preferred to those residing outside of it. The former was seen by the research-ers as 'typical' residents, who were experienced and were knowledgeable about issues faced by the communities. Thus, they were viewed as likely not only to represent their communities well but also to hold researchers to account. One HIV study CAB member said: 'when you go for interviews … they also want to find out how long you have lived in this community and how much you are known and also how respected you are in the community' (male, CAB member, HIV study).

Another criterion for researchers' selection of CAB members was people's knowledge of health-re-lated issues. Understandably, the researchers considered knowledge of HIV and TB to be important given the nature of the respective studies. Some CAB members themselves said that members must wield influence in the community for people to listen and respect them, and one factor contributing to their influence was their health-related knowledge. However, concerns were raised by residents about the bias and favouritism in the selection of CAB members, with some people alleging that volunteers in good standing with health facility management and Neighbourhood Health Committees were often picked.

The nature of CAB–community–researcher interactions

Interactions with community members

CABs performed several interfacing roles with the study communities. These included facilitating consultation and entry of the studies into the community (HIV study CAB), educating and sensitising communities about the studies and supporting recruitment and retention activities. Because the HIV study CAB was functional before the study started, it could assist researchers in organising the initial community consultation meetings. This was not the case for the TB study as its CAB was created after the study had already commenced. Instead, the Neighbourhood Health Committee played the role of a CAB until the official CAB was created. The TB study was also incidentally stopped early and all community engagement activities were consequently halted, even though the reasons for halting the study were not revealed. CAB members said researchers disrespected the community by not consulting and telling them the decision in good time.

The CABs conducted community meetings, one-on-one or door-to-door campaigns and used drama to disseminate information and educate residents about the studies. They also obtained feedback from residents using the above activities. For instance, in the HIV study, some residents questioned the scientific merits of excluding HIV-negative individuals and adjacent communities who, in their opinion, also had a high HIV burden.

Despite CAB involvement in sensitisation (information giving and education) activities, findings from interviews with key informants showed that there was low awareness among residents of the existence of CABs. However, some people knew the CAB members from their other pre-existing roles in the community. This low awareness was in part because CAB members and their representative role was never explained during research specific community sensitisation meetings.

Both CABs said that the researchers told them not to directly contact study participants. The main reason was not to compromise participants' privacy and confidentiality. A further reason was that this could constitute a conflict of interest and expose the CAB members to risk of violence in the event of a backlash against the studies. The CAB members expressed reservations about this guiding rule that were both pragmatic and ethical. Regarding the former, they felt that the ability to visit study participants would improve retention substantially. Regarding the latter, they felt that contact would enable them to understand the challenges participants experience so that they were in a better position to speak on their behalf. In any case, it was impossible to prevent some degree of contact between CAB members and study participants because they were familiar to each other through the CAB members' membership of other Community-Based Organisations. Moreover, in the HIV study, when it became clear that they were not going to meet their recruitment targets in time, researchers authorised direct contact with potential participants by asking the CAB to conduct sensitisation activities among patients at the Anti-retroviral Therapy (ART) and Tuberculosis (TB) departments, some of whom they later met at the study recruitment offices.

Interacting with researchers

The main channels through which the researchers and CABs interacted were the following: scheduled CAB meetings, ad hoc meetings (e.g. to review study material), training sessions, conferences outside the country and joint community sensitisation meetings. CAB meetings were the foremost channel for communicating issues raised by the community to researchers. The meetings in the TB study were infrequent and were stopped following suspension of the research. The HIV study CAB, however, held regular monthly meetings. Researchers were invited to provide study updates relating to the recruitment and retention of study participants, allowing the CAB to monitor the study's performance. Even though the HIV study provided regular updates relating to recruitment and retention, CAB members and the general community did not have access to critical study progress reports such as the Data Safety Monitoring Board (DSMB) reports.

CAB members felt that protocol development and review ought to be one of their most important responsibilities. However, the TB study CAB participated in neither because it was created once the study was already underway, while the HIV study CAB's involvement was limited to responding to a set of predetermined questions. However, both CABs were involved in reviewing Information Education Communications materials. The HIV study CAB also reviewed the Audio Computer Assisted Interview and suggested shortening the programme as well as including captions in local language. CAB members also identified scientific language in study documents that would be a barrier to communication and meaningful CAB involvement.

Power dynamics

Power can manifest in different forms. In this article, 'power over' and 'structural power' are used to contextualise the power imbalances and therefore the accountability relationships which existed between the community, the CABs and the researchers. 'Power over' refers to decision-making models which are characterised by control of one actor over the other (Berger, 2005). Structural power refers to institutional practices which may facilitate or hinder the action of different actors. In general, possession of knowledge about research and health by CAB members was seen as a source of power over community members as one TB study CAB member indicated: 'the difference is there, because those who are in the community have no knowledge compared to me who comes to the clinic (health facility) and learns from the researchers. So knowledge is the difference', (female, CAB member, TB study).

In fact, in reference to the influence CAB members had over the community, a key informant (opinion leader) equated the CAB's influence to that of a village headman: 'they have strong powers; they are like village headmen' (male, key informant, TB study). However, most residents did not know most CAB members as CAB members but as volunteers in different capacities. When community members understood which residents were CAB members and which other volunteer roles they had in the community, they viewed them as influential. The existence of the studies therefore offered CAB members new opportunities for attaining power and social status that are comparable to traditional forms of authority.

Additionally, proximity to researchers and health facilities was seen by CAB members as giving them an advantage over other community members. Being volunteers and being found within the health facility meant that CAB members were always in the communication loop regarding forthcoming projects, studies and other opportunities. They were not shy to enquire from researchers for such opportunities. Some of them even asked for work. Therefore, some CAB members used the CAB as a conduit for other opportunities. As one CAB member indicated, even though the initial motivation for joining the CAB might be altruism, some CAB members soon began to ask for incentives, partly driven by the demands put upon them as members.

CAB members also said 'they had potential power over researchers and they could wield it if prompted to'. According to them, an important source of their power was being resident in the area and their membership of social networks within the communities. They claimed they could use this power to influence community opinion about research if they were unsure about the benefit of the study to the community and were concerned about the safety of participants: 'If the worse comes to the worst, we can influence people not to participate in that research because we have all the information, but we do not do that because it is for the good of society' (Female, CAB member, HIV study). Researchers, aware of these close-knit social networks believed that a rumour started by a discontented CAB member could damage the image and reputation of a study.

For several reasons the power of researchers over the CABs was often manifested in the latter's inability to challenge decisions and actions made by the researchers. Firstly, a lack of ownership and control of financial resources meant that the CABs had little backing to challenge some decisions made by researchers. The two CABs were nested within their respective studies and received organisational and logistical support from them, making the CABs dependent on the studies, with no alternative sources of funding. Consequently, they were cautious of making decisions that researchers might dislike. One community member, reflecting upon the material inequalities, said that: 'in a partnership, the one with more resources has an advantage over the one without' (male, key informant, TB study).

The second reason why the CAB members were often unable to challenge researchers was the asymmetry in knowledge and technical expertise. As already mentioned, CAB members were seen to be more knowledgeable than the residents. However, CAB members themselves said that their knowledge did not compare to that of the researchers. Although no CAB member cited actual situations in which they failed to challenge decisions made by researchers due to power disparities, perceptions such as: 'someone who has more knowledge than you have can cheat you without you even knowing' (female, CAB member HIV study) attest to the influence of the power disparities between the two. Some community members even suggested researchers might exploit research participants: 'you (researchers) who have money want those people who do not have money (the community) to participate in the research so that you get the information that you want' (male, key informant, TB study).

Researchers also wielded structural power. Power asymmetry was written into the CAB guidelines (although only the HIV study CAB had such guidelines). The guidelines stipulated the roles and responsibilities for the CAB and its members. Yet the guidelines were almost exclusively targeted at the organisational arrangement of the CAB and the conduct of its members for the purpose of sensitising and communicating study related information. Nothing about the conduct of researchers or how the CAB could deal with misconduct by researchers was mentioned in the document. These guidelines reflected the concern that CAB members would use their considerable influence (discussed above) to disrupt research and jeopardise a systematic approach to data collection. For instance, in addition to the guidelines, HIV CAB members were made to sign a confidentiality note which asked them to make a strong commitment to research. There was no corresponding document for the researchers to sign that could enable them to be held accountable beyond the protocol and the ethical review process. In one CAB meeting, HIV CAB members accused researchers of only 'recognising' them (in the more general sense of engaging with them) only when they needed help. Perhaps the most flagrant disrespect encountered was when researchers failed to forewarn the TB study CAB members about the suspension of the study.

These considerations played out in the day-to-day conduct of CAB-related activities. At all times, the researchers held the 'power of approval'. They determined the type of activities CAB members conducted in the community by reviewing work plans and monitoring field activities. Researchers also had significant control over the information that was relayed in the community. One CAB member for the HIV study believed that researchers sometimes lacked confidence and trust in the CAB. He viewed the researchers' insistence on reviewing and approving messages CAB members were to disseminate in the community as an attempt to hold back information that researchers thought would be confusing and compromise recruitment efforts. This CAB member's view was supported by the fact that the HIV study coordinator said that the study was cautious with information shared in open and stakeholder meetings, especially if a possible misunderstanding was perceived.

Discussion

This paper has explored the relationship between researchers, CAB members and communities in the context of two research projects, focusing in particular on the role played by CABs. Three layers of accountability relationships were identified, namely the relationship between CABs and the community, between CABs and researchers and between the researchers and the community.

The CAB and community accountability relationship

A weak accountability relationship existed between the CAB and community mainly because residents did not directly participate in the selection of CAB members. In fact, researchers' influence on the selection process resulted in the exclusion of some interest groups such as young people. Residents accused researchers of bias and favouritism. Whilst other studies in sub-Saharan Africa suggest that it is a common practice for researchers to select CAB members (e.g. Marsh, Kamuya, Rowa, Gikonyo, & Molyneux, 2008), non-direct involvement of residents in the election of their representatives erodes the basis for the representatives' authority and legitimacy (Reddy, Buchanan, Sifunda, James, & Naidoo, 2010). This study suggests that a major challenge arising from the use of CABs was how residents could claim accountability from representatives whose existence they knew little about and in whose election they did not directly participate. Indeed, democratic elections are an important means by which people delegate their powers to representatives (Harrington, 2012; Reddy et al., 2010), thereby legitimising the authority of the elected (Judge, 1999). Lack of elections (and thus legitimacy) limited the CABs accountability to the community. With CAB members selected as they were however, the CABs were far more visible to researchers as the 'accessible face of community' (Gaventa, 2004) than to the residents who they were supposedly representing. This contrasted with CAB members who perceived their main role as the bridge between researchers and the community (including study participants), linking both ends of the relationship and thus ensuring a symmetrical accountability relationship between the two.

Moreover, researchers expressly denied CAB members permission to directly contact research partici-pants (initially, at least) and to take an active part in other study activities. Such demands by community representatives to have an active role in the conduct of research were not unique to this study. Kamuya, Marsh, Kombe, Geissler, and Molyneux (2013) reported that community representatives often wanted to take on 'a more proactive role including holding community outreach activities, accompanying field workers to participants' homes and being informed of all studies and participants in each area' (Kamuya et al., 2013). These observations shed light upon a dissonance between the intrinsic goals of commu-nity engagement as an empowering and participatory process and the reality in which community engagement often serves instrumental purposes (Simwinga et al., 2016).

The CAB and researchers' accountability relationship

The CAB and researchers interacted in several forums including CAB meetings, training, and com-munity sensitisation meetings. However, this interaction and relationship was imbalanced in favour of researchers who were more knowledgeable, more skilful and better resourced. This allowed the researchers to define the relationship with the CAB at the expense of the latter. For instance, they justified the decision to deny CAB members access to study participants using the ethical argument for privacy and confidentiality even though this presented the best opportunity to CAB members to be more answerable to the community. They also ensured that the CAB guidelines required the CAB members to be more accountable to research, without a corresponding requirement for researchers towards the CAB and the community.

However, opportunities for researchers to improve their accountability to the CAB and the commu-nity existed. Firstly, researchers acknowledged the instrumental role the CABs played in implementing ethical and high-quality research by supporting the recruitment and retention processes of the study. Secondly, they also acknowledged the CABs influence on both the community and researchers. The CABs Influence on researchers arose from their knowledge of community dynamics, their membership of close-knit social networks and their social status. As Stoecker (2013) has observed, the power of community members manifests not only in their knowledge of the community but also in numbers and relationships. Instead of embracing these positive CAB attributes, researchers were wary of the possible detrimental effects on the studies if CAB members became discontented and used the same attributes against research. For example, withdrawing their support for studies or starting rumours about the studies. In reality, the CABs' ability to carry through any threat was undermined by their dependence on researchers for financial and institutional support. Researchers need to more explicitly acknowledge the instrumental role that CABs play in research to cultivate mutual respect and trust. This could improve not only the accountability relationship between them but also increase the likelihood that CABs will perform more intrinsic roles in future research conducted by the research institutions implementing the two studies (Tindana et al., 2015).

Reflecting on implications on the researcher and community accountability relationship

The community was not consulted during protocol development for both the TB study and the HIV study. This limited community involvement at the protocol development stage affected the ensuing researcher–community accountability relationship in three main ways. Firstly, researchers were able to retain their traditional powers over the community which usually come with ethical and regulatory approval of the protocol: the power to decide which communities to work in, which population groups to intervene in, and what recruitment and retention strategies to use without meaningful consultation of community-based stakeholders. Secondly, and relatedly, the lack of and/or limited formative research in the studies missed an opportunity to build a stronger voice for the community. Such consultation would have helped researchers build strong community representation by identifying key community stakeholders eligible for election on the CABs (Simwinga & Kabero, 2014). Thirdly, ongoing updates about study progress were not sufficient and hindered a successful and transparent relationship between researchers and the community. While it was not expected of researchers to hold regular community meetings to provide ongoing feedback, a higher degree of transparency in CAB meetings could have been achieved, and more information beyond recruitment and retention data could have been provided. Sharing information from sources such as the Data Safety and Monitoring Board (DSMB) reports could have been important in this regard. This could have had the additional benefit of preparing CAB members for possible participation in the interpretation and dissemination of final study results (see also Mott, Crawford, & Group, 2008).

Conclusion

The two CABs in the research studies had a less well-defined relationship with community members and research participants than they had with researchers. This was mainly because they were not directly elected by residents and researchers prevented them from interacting with research participants. This eroded the basis for their legitimacy and their claim on research accountability. In spite of this, CABs had subtle powers over community members and researchers. They were highly regarded in the community because of their knowledge of research and health-related issues and because of their close association with researchers. Researchers too had a high regard for the CABs because of their influence in the community. Lack of inclusion and inadequate scientific knowledge and financial power still, however, made the CABs intractably weak. The CABs remained reliant on researchers for organisational, financial and logistical support. In essence, they were appendages to research studies to which they increasingly became more accountable while at the same time becoming less accountable to those they were supposed to represent. The 'interface' role that the two CABs occupied between researchers and communities was therefore considerably more unidirectional (with the CAB being accountable more to researchers than to communities) than its portrayal in bioethical literature. Such an unequal power dynamic in favour of researchers is far from ideal for research, especially while trying to promote the ideals of engagement, transparency, respect, trust and accountability.

Acknowledgements

We thank all CAB members for the TB and HIV studies for their participation in the study and Constance Mackworth-Young for useful comments and insights she provided.

Disclosure statement

No potential conflict of interest was reported by the authors.

Funding

This work was supported by the Commonwealth Scholarship Commission (CSC).

References

Becker, A. B., Israel, B. A., Gustat, J., Reyes, A. G., & Allen III, A. J. (2013). Strategies and Techniques for Effective Group Process in CBPR Partnerships. In Israel, B. A., Eng, E., Schulz, A. J. & Parker, E. A. (Eds.) *Methods for Community-Based Participatory Research for Health* (2nd ed., pp. 69–96). San Francisco: Jossey-Bass.

Berger, B. K. (2005). Power over, power with, and power to relations: Critical reflections on public relations, the dominant coalition, and activism. *Journal of Public Relations Research, 17*(1), 5–28.

Brinkerhoff, D. W. (2004). Accountability and health systems: Toward conceptual clarity and policy relevance. *Health Policy and Planning, 19*, 371–379.

Cox, L. E., Rouff, J. R., Svendsen, K. H., Markowitz, M., & Abrams, D. I. (1998). Community advisory boards: Their role in AIDS clinical trials. *Health & Social Work, 23*, 290–297.

Dickert, N., & Sugarman, J. (2005). Ethical goals of community consultation in research. *American Journal of Public Health, 95*(7), 1123–1127.

Gaventa, J. (2004). *Representation, community leadership and participation: Citizen involvement in neighbiurhood renewal and local governance.* Brighton: Institute of Development Studies.

George, A. (2003). Using accountability to improve reproductive health care. *Reproductive Health Matters, 11*, 161–170.

Green, J., & Thorogood, N. (2009). *Qualitative methods for health research.* London: Sage.

Harrington, P. (2012). *Democracy and elections.* Kenya: Paulines Publications Africa.

Israel, B. A., Schulz, A. J., Parker, P. A., & Becker, A. B. (1998). Review of community-based research: Assessing partnership approaches to improve public health. *Annual Review of Public Health, 19*, 173–202.

Judge, D. (1999). *Representation theory and practice in Britain.* London: Routledge.

Kamuya, D. M., Marsh, V., Kombe, F. K., Geissler, P. W., & Molyneux, S. C. (2013). Engaging communities to strengthen research ethics in low-income settings: Selection and perceptions of members of a network of representatives in coastal Kenya. *Developing World Bioethics, 13*, 10–20.

Liamputtong, P., & Ezzy, D. (2005). *Qualitative research methods.* Victoria: Oxford University Press.

Macqueen, K. M., Kerry, M., Alleman, P., Mcclain Burke, H., & Mack, N. (2006). *Partnering for care in the HIV prevention trials network.* Carolina: Family Health International.

MacQueen, K., Bhan, A., Frohlich, J., Holzer, J., & Sugarman, J. (2015). Evaluating community engagement in global health research: The need for metrics. *BMC Medical Ethics, 16*(1), 1–9.

Marsh, V., Kamuya, D., Rowa, Y., Gikonyo, C., & Molyneux, S. (2008). Beginning community engagement at a busy biomedical research programme: Experiences from the KEMRI CGMRC-Wellcome Trust Research Programme, Kilifi, Kenya. *Social Science & Medicine, 67*, 721–733.

Merriam, S. B. (2009). *Qualitative research: A guide to design and implementation.* San Francisco, CA: Wiley.

Minkler, M., Blackwell, A. G., Thompson, M., & Tamir, H. (2003). Community-based participatory research: Implications for public health funding. *American Journal of Public Health, 93*(8), 1210–1213.

Mott, L., Crawford, E., & Group. (2008). The role of community advisory boards in project Eban. *Journal of acquired immune deficiency syndromes (1999), 49*, S68.

Murray, N., & Beglar, D. (2009). *Writing dissertations and theses.* Harlow: Pearson Longman.

Newman, S. D., Andrews, J. O., Magwood, G. S., Jenkins, C., Cox, M. J., & Williamson, D. C. (2011). Community Advisory Boards in Community-Based Participatory Research: A Synthesis of Best Processes. *Preventing Chronic Disease,3*, A70.

Nguyen, V.-K. (2015). Treating to prevent HIV: Population trials and experimental societies. In W. P. Geissler (Ed.), *Para-states and medical science: Making African global health* (pp. 47–77). Durham, NC: Duke University Press.

Petryna, A. (2009). *When experiments travel: Clinical trials and the global search for human subjects.* Princeton, NJ: Princeton University Press.

Pratt, B., Lwin, K. M., Zion, D., Nosten, F., Loff, B., & Cheah, P. Y. (2015). Exploitation and community engagement: Can community advisory boards successfully assume a role minimising exploitation in international research? *Developing World Bioethics, 15*, 18–26.

Quinn, S. C. (2004). Ethics in public health research: Protecting human subjects: The role of community advisory boards. *American Journal of Public Health, 94*, 918–922.

Reddy, P., Buchanan, D., Sifunda, S., James, S., & Naidoo, N. (2010). The role of community advisory boards in health research: Divergent views in the South African experience. *SAHARA-J: Journal of Social Aspects of HIV/AIDS, 7*, 2–8.

Richards, L. (2009). *Handling qualitative data.* London: Sage.

Rottenburg, R. (2009). Social and public experiments and new figurations of science and politics in postcolonial Africa. *Postcolonial Studies, 12*, 423–440.

Silverman, D. (2011). *Qualitative research.* London: Sage.

Simwinga, M., & Kabero, C. (2014). Community engagement. In M. Krugger, P. Ndebele, & L. Horn (Eds.), *Research ethics in Africa: A resource for research ethics committees* (pp. 143–151). Cape Town: Sun Press.

Simwinga, M., Bond, V., Makola, N., Hoddinott, G., Belemu, S., White, R., ... Moore, A. (2016). Implementing community engagement for combination prevention: Lessons Learnt from the first year of the HPTN 071 (PopART) community-randomized study. *Current HIV/AIDS Reports, 13*, 194–201.

Slevin, K. W., Ukpong, M., & Heise, L. (2008). Community engagement in HIV prevention trials: Evolution of the field and opportunities for growth. *Research Gate.* January.

Stoecker, R. (2013). *Research methods for community change: A project-based approach.* Los Angeles, CA: Sage.

Strauss, R. P., Sengupta, S., Quinn, S. C., Goeppinger, J., Spaulding, C., Kegeles, S. M., & Millett, G. (2001). The role of community advisory boards: Involving communities in the informed consent process. *American Journal of Public Health, 91,* 1938–1943.

Tindana, P. O., Singh, J. A., Tracy, C. S., Upshur, R. E., Daar, A. S., Singer, P. A., … Lavery, J. V. (2007). Grand challenges in global health: Community engagement in research in developing countries. *PLoS Medicine, 4,* e273.

Tindana, P., de Vries, J., Campbell, M., Littler, K., Seeley, J., Marshall, P., … Parker, J (2015). Community engagement strategies for genomic studies in Africa: A review of the literature. *BMC Medical Ethics, 16,* e273.

Wakefield, S. (2005). Community advisory boards. In Kahn, P. (Ed.), *AIDS vaccine handbook: Global perspectives* (pp. 117). New York, NY: AIDS Vaccine Advocacy Coalition.

Woolf, S. H., Zimmerman, E., Haley, A., & Krist, A. H. (2016). Authentic engagement of patients and communities can transform research, practice, and policy. *Health Affairs, 35*(4), 590–594.

Empathic response and no need for perfection: reflections on harm reduction engagement in South Africa

Anna Versfeld, Andrew Scheibe, Shaun Shelly and Janine Wildschut

ABSTRACT

The importance of community involvement in public health research processes is well established. The literature is, however, less forthcoming about processes of community inclusion in public health project implementation, especially when it comes to projects focusing on key populations. The Step Up Project is the first multi-city harm reduction service provision project for people who inject drugs in South Africa. Since inception, the Project has made concerted efforts to work with and alongside people who actively identify as people who inject drugs. This paper outlines two features in relation to project-beneficiary dynamics that emerged in a qualitative project evaluation conducted by an external researcher and a funder representative. The first was that people accessing the project comfortably expressed criticisms of both themselves and the project, and noted when their behaviour contradicted project ideals. The second was the extent to which engagement with the project was reported to be fostering a renewed sense of personhood and right to exist in the world. These findings are, we suggest, in principle related to two forms of community engagement: consistent empathic response and community advisory groups. This implies that programmes need to focus on their mode of approach as much as on the content of their approach. It further implies that programme impact not be limited to quantitative assessment measures.

Calls for inclusion

At the 2016 International AIDS conference in Durban, South Africa 'key populations' were a centre of debate and discussion. Concerns were that the United Nations Joint Programme on HIV and AIDS (UNAIDS) 90–90–90 treatment goals[1] (2014) for the end of the AIDS epidemic will only be reached through successfully responding to the high prevalence of HIV amongst key populations, where key populations refers to those who face untenably high infection risk due to risk behaviours, stigma and discrimination, criminalising laws and insufficient service provision.[2]

Speakers and audience members at the conference called for greater inclusion of key population representatives in programme design and implementation. This was, however, something only partly achieved at the conference itself. While representation from sex workers and men who have sex with men was notably present, representation from people who use drugs was markedly lacking (Shelly, 2016) and prisoner representation was absent. Inclusion on the global stage, moreover, does not necessarily translate to inclusion on the ground. At the conference men who have sex with men and sex workers spoke of the ways in which inclusion seemed to respond to the requirements of funders, rather than the needs of the target populations. Calls were for inclusion at a country policy and local project level that went beyond tokenism.

A generous amount of literature and process guidelines provide information on how this might be achieved in research processes. (See, for example, AIDS Vaccine Advocacy Coalition (AVAC) and UNAIDS international guidelines (2011) and National Health Research Ethics Council (2012) South African Guidelines.) The literature is, however, less forthcoming about inclusion in public health *implementation* projects. In 2017, the United Nations Office on Drugs and Crime, the International Network of People Who Inject Drugs and global partners released guidance around implementing HIV and hepatitis C programmes with people who inject drugs, with an emphasis on community empowerment and participation (United National Office on Drugs and Crime et al., 2017). This paper examines the processes and results of continuous participant inclusion efforts through the Step Up Project, a demonstration harm reduction project in three cities in South Africa. Run by TB HIV Care (THC),[3] in collaboration with OUT Wellbeing.[4] The Step Up Project has provided harm reduction services to people who inject drugs since mid-2015, as one of the first, and certainly the largest, needle and syringe programmes in South Africa.

The project was set up to develop and maintain proximity with people who use drugs. Staff teams included people who use drugs. From initiation stages the Project has made concerted efforts to include 'service users' (those accessing the programme services) as active, valuable, guiding voices and to ensure that staff teams include people who used drugs. People who inject drugs were included in the formative assessment and programmatic mapping stages of the project and continued involvement through on-going community advisory group (CAG) processes, which are described elsewhere (Scheibe et al., 2017). Here we, a group of harm reduction advocates involved either in setting up the project or in evaluating it, look at the successes, limitations and lessons we can draw from this demonstration project related to such inclusion. We draw on a qualitative evaluation process conducted six months after the initiation of needle and syringe services, and a year after the formative assessment.

We started the evaluation doubtful that the service user participants would provide critical feedback. People who use drugs generally have few incentives to reveal their worlds to researchers who are, as we were, passing through. Consequently, researchers often end up gathering fabrications (Bourgois, 1995). Indeed, during this research we heard about how people who inject drugs were schooling each other on the narratives that would allow them access to the research process (and related remuneration) being undertaken by another local NGO. Long-term ethnographic immersion is one method used to gain insights into lived experience and the differences between what is said and what is done. As evaluators, however, our engagements were short, and pointed, while the project under discussion was set to stay. Moreover, the fact that one evaluator was from a funder organisation could have raised fears that admissions of less than perfect implementation would result in future funding cuts.

Harm reduction also relies – at least to some extent – on the presentation of people who use drugs as self-regulating, responsible and responsive subjects, who will, as far as possible, act in rational ways to maximise their own health possibilities. The emphasis on individual people who inject drugs as capable of (and responsible for) care for self and others has been part of a larger neoliberal trend in which responsibility for health and welfare was devolved from the state towards the individual (Moore & Fraser, 2006). While this heralds a notable shift away from the presentation of drugs users as inherently pathological and deviant, what it means is that people who use drugs risk marking themselves as irrational and irresponsible if they acknowledge rejection or only partial adoption of harm reduction discourses and practices (Moore & Fraser, 2006). This encourages the voicing of harm reduction narratives and assertions of adherence to harm reduction principles even when uptake is, in fact, sketchy at best. Ethnographers have noted that people who inject drugs have tended to assert themselves as enacting the ideals of harm reduction projects, while their actions have indicated otherwise. For example, individuals might claim the habitual use of bleach, while openly not doing so (Campbell & Shaw, 2008); or claim never sharing needles, in contradiction to the reports of injecting partners (Maher, 2002), and without mentioning sharing habits within trust relationships that they do not deem risky (Rhodes, Davis, & Judd, 2004). We, however, found that while participants were well aware of the behaviours the project was designed to elicit, they provided us with nuanced responses – neither unremittingly positive nor negative – about their own drug use and the project implementation.

The responses we received could be read, and explained in a number of ways. They could be a happy result of the ways in which the evaluators piggybacked on the trust developed through the long-term relations developed by project staff, especially as staff themselves had either historical or present drug use habits and were therefore to some extent insiders. They could also be a result of project staff efforts to implement a 'bottom-up' harm reduction approach (Marlatt, 1996) in which service users were actively consulted in project planning and implementation. This approach could have set the expectation that the 'ideal' service user (from the perspective of those implementing the project) was a 'responsibilised' service user – one who accepted accountability for their own health and health choices (Robins, 2006). Read this way the nuanced responses we describe below are related to complex power dynamics of health care practice (Mol, 2008), the governmentality of harm reduction implementation, and the positionality of the evaluators.

These approaches are valuable, but ours is a different task. Cognisant of how frequently people who use drugs are not regarded as the experts on their own lives we take an ethnographic (and moral) approach of presenting peoples' words and worlds as they were presented to us. We also write as researcher-practitioners committed to developing texts that are legible to (and verifiable by) the people we write about. In this, we suggest that the responses we found were related to the ways in which the consistent empathic responses of the project team combined with the regular CAG meetings regenerated a sense of self and right to influence the world around them in the service users.

Evaluation as method

This paper draws largely on the findings of a qualitative evaluation of project activities that took place in February and March 2016, approximately eight months after project initiation. The evaluation, as described by the research protocol, sought to assess 'the feasibility and acceptability of providing a package of HIV prevention and harm reduction services for people who inject drugs in Cape Town, Durban and Pretoria'. In this the primary focus was assessment of programme implementation possibilities. Assessment of the uptake and impact of the services was a secondary focus.

We used a standardised process of data collection in each of the three project sites. This included three days' participant observation of outreach and office operations; two feedback sessions with service users; one feedback session with stakeholders; and four interviews with project team members. A total of 55 project service users, 15 stakeholders and 12 staff were included in the evaluation. Efforts were made to gather a cross-representation of perspectives. This meant including – as far as possible – a representative sample of service users by race, age and gender, something that differed by city (see below). This, to some extent, reflected the limitations of the project. White males were over-represented. Foreign nationals and women were under-represented. The prior because they reportedly avoided the project due to fears they would be asked for their papers; the latter likely a combination of the lesser number of women injecting and (reportedly) limitations placed on their movements by their male partners. A further study limitation lies in the fact that we did not ask individuals to self-identify race. We can therefore only speak in broad brush-strokes about race, and do not link quotes to race.

Participant feedback sessions were divided into two groups per site. One group was comprised of participants who were regularly part of the CAG processes (see below). The other included service users who were not actively involved in CAG processes. This separation was set up to avoid the possible stifling of more critical voices from the participants who felt increased loyalty to the project through their greater involvement.

Reimbursements of R50 (approximately $3) were provided for participation to cover the costs of time lost to income generating activities. Written consent was obtained from all participants. Ethical clearance for these processes was obtained from the University of the Western Cape Research Ethics Committee. Data was were coded and analysed in Nvivo.

Step Up: a process of daily engagement

At the time of the evaluation, the Step Up Project was providing services to almost 1500 people across the three cities. This is a small percentage of the estimated total 67,000 (Petersen, Myers, van Hout, Plüddemann, & Parry, 2013) people who inject drugs in the country. This, in turn is a small percentage of total drug users. In South Africa drugs are more frequently inhaled, even in the case of heroin, the most commonly injected drug (Dada et al., 2016).

In each city, the profile of the population of people who use drugs differed. The Cape Town and Durban sites largely provided services to people who had long histories of injecting drug use, the majority of whom were white.[5] Cape Town had the largest (though still small) representation of methamphetamine injectors. The Pretoria site, in contrast, largely served people who had transitioned from smoking to injecting heroin in recent years, most of whom were black. In all cities, however, white participants were disproportionately represented in CAG groups.[6] The project was adapted to city particularities, such as the (very variable) relationships between the drug using community and law enforcement; the locations where drugs are bought and injected; and organisational infrastructure influences such as team size and available resources. However, all approaches were underscored with a harm reduction ethos and daily activities were similar across the cities.

Daily activities

In three cities across South Africa, on four mornings a week, small teams of outreach workers, including a nurse, a counsellor, peer educators (outreach workers with social links to the populations served) and a driver, prepared their stocks and supplies for the day. The nurse would work from the mobile clinic or a gazebo providing – amongst other things – HIV counselling and testing, tuberculosis screening, and wound care. Daily stocks included sterile injecting equipment (needles and syringes, alcohol swabs and sterile water); wound care supplies; condoms (male and female); lubricant; a model dildo and vagina (for demonstration purposes) and documents to use in education processes.

Daily routes were influenced by the formative assessment process and reshaped based on input from the CAG processes (Scheibe et al., 2017) to reach the maximum possible number of potential service users over a week period. Some – especially those asking for money at traffic intersections – were reached through whistle-stop service delivery at their regular pitches. On seeing a recognised figure, the team would pull the van up on the side of the road, ask how they are doing; check on any injuries or wounds they knew the person to have; and collect used needles and provide sterile injecting equipment. A few minutes later the team would move on. In other places, where more service users congregated, the driver would park the mobile clinic or car in a set location and settle in for half an hour, or more. Some of the project team would stay to serve those who came on seeing, or hearing about, the team's arrival. Other team members fanned out in groups of two or more for safety, seeking people in the surrounding areas. They were to be found in the far corners of parks and areas of bush, in underpasses and under bridges, and in sprawling buildings that had not seen sanitation or running water in years; the places where they lived and kept themselves – as far as possible – dry and out of sight of often less than obliging law officials. (Harassment, including confiscation of injecting equipment, both sterile and used; extortion; assaults and detention without cause, a continual part of life for many people who use drugs.) They were also to be found in the broad open spaces of public life such as transport hubs and central city streets; places where business, theirs included, was conducted.

For the most part the project teams displayed a carefully balanced combination of haste and patience. Sterile needles were quickly dispatched when queues developed, or when a service user was edgy and impatient in the throes of withdrawal. At other times programme teams settled into languid chats, or detailed, unhurried health discussions and education processes. On a street corner in Durban, a conversation stretched into half an hour as a peer educator explained how female condoms could be used to sex workers' advantage. The peer's offer had been met by refusal, accompanied by laughter and the shake of an armful of bracelets made of the outer rubber ring of unused female condoms from the leader of the group. After the discussion extra condoms had to be fetched from the van.

At another site, two peers walked along an abandoned railway track picking up discarded needles, while another sat in the back of the van providing sterile needle and syringe packs. The nurse sat in the front of the van attending to a seeping wound on the hand of a man, in his mid-thirties, who spoke of his troubles while his wound was attended to. Softly weeping, he spoke of past traumas and his deep depression. 'Who do you talk to [about these things]?' asked the nurse, gently. 'I'm talking to you,' replied her patient. 'We're not here very often …' reflected the nurse. '[Then] I don't talk to anyone …' Conversations such as this, steeped in sadness, were abundant. But we also witnessed interactions that were jocular – a wide smile and a double thumbs-up as the mobile clinic passed; a wave and a jaunty call of 'I'm coming now!' from someone heading to fetch their stash of used needles before coming to get new sterile injecting equipment.

The team's days passed in these ways: seeking out people who inject drugs in places they were known to live and frequent, supply provision, conversations, health check-ins, education processes, and HIV counselling and testing processes. They would also collect details on human rights abuses; noting them down on site to later feed them into a database for advocacy purposes. At the end of each day they returned to their offices, to fill in their paper work and undertake any immediate office-based duties that had arisen from the day.

Unscripted responses

Summerson Carr (2010) has noted how particular, scripted, ways talking about addiction in treatment centres can become so inculcated that they shape all interactions between those seeking and providing treatment. Others, as we indicated above, have noted that people who use drugs have few incentives to provide researchers with anything but what they are seeking to hear (Bourgois, 1995), or to report critically on their actual uptake of harm reduction practices (Campbell & Shaw, 2008; Maher, 2002; Rhodes et al., 2004).

Our experience was different. For the most part service user participants in the evaluation indicated that their engagement with Step Up resulted in behaviour changes in line with the aims of the imple-mentation staff. They reported, for example, that prior to the project needles were rented, shared and/ or used for very extended periods, and that this had changed. 'I remember when [before this service] I had to use a needle, probably for a month … one needle. You know sometimes you can't buy a needle …' said one man in his late forties. 'I know when there weren't needles around … It was so scary to me. You would see three people on one needle. I don't see that anymore! I don't see anybody sharing a needle anymore. And that is a relief to me' said another participant. But we, the evaluators, were also provided with notably more tempered responses. Across the sites, service users indicate that sharing and reusing of needles was greatly reduced, but that to some extent it continued. 'I think before the CAG meetings we were buying our own needles, so we were using them more than once, now that we are getting our needles for free, *most of us* are using them once then throwing them away,' said one beneficiary. Another explained, 'Before [it was like], "Okay, you want a needle, here's a needle", but now we don't give a [used] needle *just like that.*' And a man in his mid twenties explained that, '*We are sup-posed to* be one needle one shot … [but] sometimes I use my needle more than once, because I can't carry three or four needles with me if I am going to make four shots in [a particular location] so I take one needle with me, and I swap that at the end of the day'. Service user participants further indicated that they knew that the project advocated for the use of alcohol swabs to clean the patch of skin where they were about to inject to avoid infections at the injecting site, but most indicated that they did not bother with this. They also reported their use of sterile water to be limited.

These departures from the project ideals seemed to be partly due to participants not fully understand-ing the relevance of the ideal actions. But they were also explained to us in terms of life practicalities.

Carrying needles (sterile or used) – especially in numbers that could not be easily concealed – held a risk of arrest because needles could be used by law enforcement as proof of drug use. 'I'm not going to walk around with 21 needles in my bag. If they catch me they will throw away the key!' Explained one woman, in her fifties. Injecting in a public space has to be done quickly to lower the risk of being caught by law enforcement. Swabbing takes additional time, raising the risk of being caught by law enforcement.

Desperation in times of withdrawal was cited as another reason for not following ideal practice. 'When you're [withdrawing] you don't care!' said one participant. Another, Jason, explained that he knew he should use different injecting sites on his body, but that in the mornings, when he was withdrawing,

I always use this vein, because … I don't know if this whole vein is blown … I don't even have to aim, I just push the needle in and the blood comes out. Later I change [veins]. Your veins seem to run away when you have [are withdrawing].

Laziness and impatience were other reasons provided.

I'm lazy to look for a vein, and the situation that I'm in, where I'm doing it, you have to be very fast because of being caught, so I always use this vein, it is there at all times. It is quick, I am gone.

Jen, a woman in her twenties spent most of the session semi-asleep on her partner's shoulder, but she pepped up for occasional comments such as 'I don't use swabs at all!' She explained this lack of use saying (with an unapologetic shrug), 'I'm just impatient'.

Service user participants were, then openly critical of the practicalities of the project ideals and of their own willingness to be bothered with following what they knew to be actions that limited the possible risks to their own health. They also admitted that they sometimes manipulated the service provision staff. Moreover, though they were very largely positive about the role the project staff played in their lives at one site a staff member was described as 'miserable, rude, hostile, and stigmatising' and having 'no qualms about [not] hiding her disdain for addicts …'.[7] She explained the alternative course of action she took: She would break the tip of the needle and throw this in a bush and put the rest of the needle and the syringe in a municipal bin. Throwing the needle tip in a bush was her way of reducing the chances that municipal workers would get a needle stick injury when they emptied the bins. By her own reckoning, she was behaving as ethically as possible given the constraints of her life conditions and the risks of law enforcement.

We saw, then, that the service user participants in our evaluation were not, as might be expected from the literature, positioning themselves as ethical beings through presenting themselves as consistently enacting the behaviours the project required of them. Rather, they were positioning themselves as ethical actors through admitting that they, to some degree, were not acting on project ideals.

There are likely multiple reasons for these responses. We suspect that the attitudes, approach, origin and knowledge base of the evaluators were contributing factors. Both were white women and did not have histories that linked them to the participants, but they did have extensive experience working with people who use drugs and were therefore not shocked or surprised at revelations about some of the grittier details of life. Their presence and engagement were, moreover endorsed by the Step Up Project team members, which – given appreciation of the project – would have provided an immediate level of credibility. They also set up the room to level power dynamics, with the participants and one researcher sitting on chairs in a circle and the other facilitator sitting on the floor in the middle making notes on large sheets of newsprint for all to see. As the participants looked on they were able to correct any errors, and make suggestions about additional important information they felt needed inclusion. Ease was likely enhanced by the fact that the spaces used were familiar to the participants as they were used for other events run by the Step Up Project. Given the extent of stigma and marginalisation faced (and described) by the participants it is, however, unlikely that it was the research environment alone that fostered the nature of the responses we received. Drawing on the explanations provided by the participants themselves, we suggest that the key contributing factors lay in two aspects of the project implementation: empathic responsiveness and CAG processes.

Empathic response: 'You *are* somebody'

During the evaluation, each feedback session started with the evaluators asking what services the participants had received from the Step Up Project. Most that were described were those we expected: the receipt of needle packs; HIV and tuberculosis testing; information and learning (on, for example, safer injecting and overdose prevention); referral and accompaniment to health care services; and commodities such as condoms, lubrication and hygiene packs, which, at a minimum consisted of a toothbrush, toothpaste and soap. In addition to these expected planned services, less tangible, but equally – if not more – valued services were reported in all feedback sessions. These included presence, listening, counselling and the general feeling of being cared for. 'They're always here for us,' said one young woman in Cape Town. 'Since the project started … we have friends now. If you need someone to go and talk to, you have someone who really cares and understands where you are, where you are coming from,' said a participant from Pretoria. In Durban, we were told how the project staff kept a register of service users' closest family members, so that the family would be informed in case of death. That they would not die without the knowledge of their families was provided as an example of the depth of care they received. Also in Durban, but in a different feedback session, the way the staff went looking for service users, seeking them out where they knew they were likely to be was cited as an example of care. 'How does that make you feel?' we asked. 'That makes you feel like you are *somebody*,' explained an older man, going on to say, tentatively, 'My family rejected me, so … but you *are* somebody.'

The Project's focus on human rights further contributed to a sense of personal value. Recorded violations were compiled into reports to use in advocacy efforts; education processes taught people exactly what the legalities were of their everyday behaviours, from carrying injecting paraphernalia, to living on the street, to begging for money. The teams also engaged with law enforcement and health care professionals, sensitising them to the needs and rights of people who use drugs in a climate where drug use is criminalised, almost all interventions have been abstinence-based, and there is a limited openness to harm reduction. Those on the receiving end of services were not always aware of the intricacies of these activities, but many were, broadly speaking, aware of these interactions (which sometimes verged on battles). As a participant explained,

> They are really trying to get police and the community on board, to see that it is about sickness … they are not encouraging us to use drugs, but trying to prevent us from getting HIV and hep[atitis] C sicknesses and they are trying to get the police and metro police to jump on board with them.

Together, the experience of being looked for, listened to, advocated on behalf of, and provided for gave service users the grounded sense of 'you matter'.

The regeneration of sense of self as a valuable entity was placed in the context of the daily erosion of self-confidence, shaped not only by rejection from families and mainstream society. 'Because we are users, people see us different[ly]. They look down on us … they think we are dogs,' explained one participant in Durban. Jill, a woman in her mid-fifties, added to the discussion, 'As a user you lose confidence and self-esteem with the public, especially when you are "hustling" (panhandling) and people are rejecting you all day, you start feeling like shit.'

What the participants were describing as 'care' was less about the practical provisions of commodities such as sterile injecting equipment (though this featured) and far more about consistent empathic response. As one team leader said, they had developed relationships through 'treating everyone like humans' and through responding to the needs of those accessing services, whether they are within the scope of the work, or not. Another, similarly, explained, 'If someone is in big trouble, we'll go.' He described a situation in which they were notified that a beneficiary was hit by a car, and, though it was late at night, they went to find him and take him to the hospital. 'That builds a lot of credibility.' He further said, that developing trust was largely about presenting themselves as fundamentally no different from the people they were working with. 'We know you, we understand you, we used to be you', was the message the project implementers sought to give.

Empathic response has been highlighted in the literature as the key element of effective substance use treatment processes. It has been shown to be even more important in improving treatment outcomes that the type of therapeutic response (Ashton & Witton, 2004; Miller & Miller, 2009; Miller & Moyers, 2015). The Step Up teams were not trying to engage people in treatment, but their manner of engagement made people feel like they mattered and their experiences and opinions had value. It seems likely that this affirmation of personhood played into the ways in which service users responded to our questions and probing with responses that did not necessarily cast them, or the project, in the best of light. It is also likely that the norm created by the project of empathic response spilled over onto us, the researchers, and it was therefore assumed that critical engagement would be received without judgement.

Community advisory groups

'Community Advisory Boards' (of which CAGS are one form) are a popular way of undertaking community engagement in large-scale health research processes. Their capacity to reduce exploitation in researched communities is not uncontested (see Pratt et al., 2015), but they have been shown to assist through providing a place of negotiation between researchers and participants (Morin et al., 2008). In South Africa, the National Health Research Ethics Committee (NHREC) guidelines (2012) provide a framework for how this should be done. However, as with inclusion processes in general, there has been limited information as to how this approach can be integrated into service delivery, rather than research, activities.[8]

CAGs have been integral to the way in which the Step Up Project has been set up and run. They grew out of stakeholder engagement processes conducted in each city during formative assessment processes whereby locations frequented by people who use drugs were mapped, health needs were outlined and numbers were estimated (Scheibe et al., 2017). Subsequently, they have been run on at least a monthly basis in each city. Fundamentally designed to elicit project input, involvement was minimally reimbursed with R40 ($2.40) per session to encourage participation despite time lost for income generation.[9] As the project progressed the purpose of CAGs started to transmute. Rather than being a place where service users provided input to strengthen project implementation, CAGs started to be a forum for the dissemination of information to service users.

In the feedback sessions, we found that participants who were involved in the CAG meetings found these to be so integral to their experience of the project, that they were unable to discuss outreach services without relating them to the CAG processes. Some participants indicated that the reimbursements held diminishing importance the longer they participated. 'At first I came for the money, afterwards I came and I met a lot of people, I learned a lot of stuff and the more I came the more I want to be here …' said one man in Cape Town. Others went so far as to question whether reimbursements should be provided at all given that they saw themselves as receiving, rather than providing, a service. Given the continuous, daily drive to obtain enough money to maintain drug use, and the fact that the CAG meetings took away time that was described as usually used for income generation, this was an exceptional offer, and not one agreed to by all the participants.

As with continuous empathic responses, CAGs were reported to provide a space for the growth of community and the renewal of a sense of self. Amin, a man in his twenties, reflected,

> If you live a life like ours, you start to see yourself as less than nothing, but here we started to give back some meaning to life and that we also count, we realised that we have rights just because we are also human.

And Jill explained,

> They are there as a back-up. It gives me a little bit of empowerment. I am a bit empowered, knowing that there is someone behind me that is not looking down on me. Before I came to the CAG meetings I was quite depressed. Now I know it is okay if someone rejects me, because I know I have my backup and my family.

The 'family' and 'backup' Jill was referring to was her fellow CAG members.

The ways in which the CAG meetings have resulted in the strengthening of a sense of community amongst service users, and a renewed individual sense of being care-worthy seems to have been the result of the regularity of the meetings which brought people (service users and providers) together.

The development of group solidarity and newly constituted social networks has been documented else-where in randomised control trial processes (Morin et al., 2008) and in HIV implementation programmes (see, for example, Nguyen, Ako, & Niamba, 2007). Here, we suggest that a further, inadvertent, result of the CAG processes may have been that the dialogue developed in these processes enabled service users to feel they had a right (and perhaps even a duty) to engage critically with programme provision.

Conclusion

Step Up Project participants asserted themselves as ethical beings through their critical engagement of both their own behaviours and the services provided. We have suggested in this paper that this was largely fostered through a combination of consistent empathic responsiveness of the project staff and the active efforts to generate participant feedback through CAG processes. We want to stress in closing that in saying that the critical responses we received from service user participants was unexpected we do not mean to imply that we expected dishonesty from people who use drugs. Rather, it is to say that we recognised that there were a number of motives for the less than forthright responses to an evaluation processes set up and undertaken by harm reduction advocates, such as ourselves. These include the ways in which harm reduction relies on the presentation of individuals who will do all they can to maximise their health given the opportunities; the short-term nature of the relationship between the evaluators and the service user participants; and the desires service users may have had to provide positive narrative about the people providing them with essential supplies, especially as one of the evaluators was from a funder organisation.

Harm reduction implementation programmes generally seek to impact on health-related behaviours to improve health outcomes. These outcomes tend to be narrowly defined in relation to a measureable reduction in morbidity and mortality. The Step Up Project qualitative evaluation findings, however, indicate that when harm reduction implementation is done in a way that develops engagement – both in everyday interactions of health care provision and in the more structured environment of CAGs – standardised, easily measureable health outcomes may be accompanied by more subtle, but equally important outcomes for service users: the (re) generation of the sense of a right to exist, comment on and shape the world they live in. Our findings, then, provide a different perspective to the literature that indicates that CAGs disproportionately serve those implementing the project (Pratt et al., 2015). They also suggest that inclusion processes need not be perfect. What is perhaps more important is the consistency of the responsiveness shown to participants and their needs. This should be an aim of intervention projects if they want their effects to be more than skin deep.

Notes

1. These UNAIDS goals are as follows,

   By 2020, 90% of all people living with HIV will know their HIV status. By 2020, 90% of all people with diagnosed HIV infection will receive sustained antiretroviral therapy. By 2020, 90% of all people receiving antiretroviral therapy will have viral suppression. (UNAIDS, 2014)

2. The South African National Strategic Plan on HIV, TB and STIs (2017–2022) includes sex workers, men who have sex with men, transgender people, people who use drugs and inmates as key populations for HIV and STIs" (South African National AIDS Council, 2017).
3. www.tbhivcare.org.
4. See www.out.org.za.
5. We delineate racial categories with the full awareness that these are constructed and contested.
6. This emerged as a critique of the project during the evaluation. It was likely due to the fact that white people living in poverty and inhabiting the city centre are quickly recognised (or cast) as people who use drugs. The early stages of the project therefore found white people who use drugs and drew on their networks to build CAGs and to find other potential participants.
7. This was dealt with subsequent to the evaluation.

8. The International Network of People Who Use Drugs has, however, recently published a practical guide for implementing HIV and hepatitis C interventions with people who use drugs, see http://www.inpud.net/en/iduit-implementing-comprehensive-hiv-and-hcv-programmes-people-who-inject-drugs.
9. The role played by reimbursements was not entirely positive. Funding limitations dictated that a limited number of participants (usually between 50 and 60 participants) could be reimbursed per meeting. This resulted in a degree of competition and gatekeeping.

Acknowledgements

We are immensely grateful to all the implementing teams and service users who shared their knowledge and experiences with us. Our thanks, too, to the management at TB HIV Care and especially Andrea Schneider, Nelson Mendeiros, Kalvanya Padayachee and Rudolph Basson for their work in running the Step Up Project and supporting the evaluation process. We further thank Mainline and the Centres for Disease Control and Prevention for their support for TB HIV Care programmes with key populations.

Disclosure statement

The authors declare no conflicts of interest.

Funding

This work was supported by the United States Centres of Disease Control and Prevention [grant number NU2GGH000257] and Mainline [grant number 15.08.03.MLN.026], [grant number BtG2 MLN PC 001].

References

Ashton, M., & Witton, J. (2004). The power of the welcoming reminder. *Drug and Alcohol Findings, 11*, 4–19.

Bourgois, P. (1995). *In search of respect: Selling crack in El Barrio*. Cambridge: Cambridge University Press.

Campbell, N. D., & Shaw, S. J. (2008). Incitements to discourse: Illicit drugs, harm reduction, and the production of ethnographic subjects. *Cultural Anthropology, 23*(4), 688–717. doi:10.1111/j.1548-1360.2008.00023.x

Carr, S. (2010). *Scripting addiction: The politics of therapeutic talk and American sobriety*. Princeton, NJ: Princeton University Press.

Dada, S., Erasmus, J., Burnhams, N. H., Parry, C., Bhana, A., Timol, F., & Fourie, D. (2016). *Monitoring alcohol, tobacco and other drug abuse treatment admission in South Africa*. South African Community Epidemiology Network on Drug Use (SACENDU).

Maher, L. (2002). Don't leave us this way: Ethnography and injecting drug use in the age of AIDS. *International Journal of Drug Policy, 13*, 311–325.

Marlatt, G. A. (1996). Harm reduction: Come as you are. *Addictive Behaviours, 21*(6), 779–788.

Miller, P. G., & Miller, W. R. (2009). What should we be aiming for in the treatment of addiction? *Addiction, 104*(5), 685–686. doi:10.1111/j.1360-0443.2008.02514.x

Miller, W., & Moyers, T. (2015). The forest and the trees: Relational and specific factors in addiction treatment. *Addiction, 110*(3), 401–413. doi:10.1111/add.12693

Mol, A. (2008). *The logic of care: Health and the problem of patient choice*. London: Routledge.

Moore, D., & Fraser, S. (2006). Putting at risk what we know: Reflecting on the drug-using subject in harm reduction and its political implications. *Social Science and Medicine, 62*(12), 3035–3047. doi:10.1016/j.socscimed.2005.11.067

Morin, S. F., Morfit, S., Maiorana, A., Aramrattana, A., Goicochea, P., Mutsambi, J. M., … Richards, T. A. (2008). Building community partnerships: Case studies of community advisory boards at research sites in Peru, Zimbabwe, and Thailand. *Clinical Trials International, 5*(2), 147–156. doi:10.1177/1740774508090211

National Health Research Ethics Council. (2012). *Guidelines for community advisory groups*. Pretoria: Medical Research Council.

Nguyen, V., Ako, C. Y., & Niamba, P. (2007). Adherence as therapeutic citizenship: Impact of the history of access to antiretroviral drugs on adherence to treatment, 31–35.

Petersen, Z., Myers, B., van Hout, M.-C., Plüddemann, A., & Parry, C. (2013). Availability of HIV prevention and treatment services for people who inject drugs: Findings from 21 countries. *Harm Reduction Journal, 10*(1), 1–7. doi:10.1186/1477-7517-10-13

Pratt, B., Lwin, K. M., Zion, D., Nosten, F., Loff, B., & Cheah, P. Y. (2015). Exploitation and community engagement: Can community advisory boards successfully assume a role minimising exploitation in international research? *Developing World Bioethics, 15*(1), 18–26. doi:10.1111/dewb.12031

Rhodes, T., Davis, M., & Judd, A. (2004). Hepatitis C and its risk management among drug injectors in London: Renewing harm reduction in the context of uncertainty. *Addiction, 99*(5), 621–633. doi:10.1111/j.1360-0443.2004.00692.x

Robins, S. (2006). From " rights" to "ritual": AIDS activism in South Africa. *American Anthropologist, 108*(2), 312–323.

Scheibe, A., Shelly, S., Lambert, A., Schneider, A., Basson, R., Medeiros, N., … Hausler, H. (2017). Using a programmatic mapping approach to plan for HIV prevention and harm reduction interventions for people who inject drugs in three South African cities. *Harm Reduction Journal, 14*(1), 35. doi:10.1186/s12954-017-0164-z

Shelly, S. (2016). How an AIDS conference sidelined an at-risk population. *Open Society Foundation*. Retrieved from https://www.opensocietyfoundations.org/voices/how-aids-conference-sidelined-risk-population

South African National AIDS Council. (2017). Let our actions count: South Africa's national strategic plan for HIV, TB and STIs 2017 – 2022. Retrieved from http://sanac.org.za/wp-content/uploads/2017/05/NSP_FullDocument_FINAL.pdf

UNAIDS, A. (2011). Good participatory practice: Guidelines for biomedical HIV prevention trials 2011. Geneva. Retrieved from http://www.unaids.org/en/resources/documents/2011/20110629_JC1853_GPP_Guidelines_2011%20OK

UNAIDS. (2014). *90-90-90 An ambitious treatment target to help end the AIDS epidemic*. Retrieved from http://www.unaids.org/en/resources/documents/2017/90-90-90

United Nations Office on Drugs and Crime, International Network of People Who Use Drugs, Joint United Nations Programme on HIV/AIDS, United Nations Development Programme, United Nations Population Fund, World Health Organization, & United States Agency for International Development. (2017). *Implementing comprehensive HIV and HCV programmes with people who inject drugs: Practical guidance for collaborative interventions*. Vienna: United Nations Office on Drugs and Crime.

Community engagement in an economy of harms: reflections from an LGBTI-rights NGO in Malawi

Crystal Biruk and Gift Trapence

ABSTRACT

Drawing on our experiences as an anthropologist and a researcher-activist working with a lesbian, gay, bisexual, transgender, and intersex (LGBTI) rights NGO in Malawi, this paper presents reflections on the ethics of engaging LGBTI-identified Malawians in research and other projects. While community engagement is normatively discussed as a tactic for creating meaningful dialogue and collaboration between researchers and the researched, this paper advocates a broadening of the term 'research' to encompass NGO work and activities with LGBTI persons in order to complicate normative discussions of harm – rooted in biomedical research or clinical trial contexts – that cast it primarily as visible bodily or mental suffering that befalls research participants. First, we discuss some less obvious risks faced by LGBTI-identified volunteer peer educators as they go about their work, and, second, we show how seemingly minor benefits such as provision of per diems for attending workshops generate patron/client relations and mostly unfulfilled expectations for future financial or other support that might be construed as a form of harm. Throughout, we emphasize how LGBTI people learn to navigate an 'economy of harms,' a network of social relations that hinge on transactions and obligations that are simultaneously risky and potentially profitable. A more capacious interpretation of harms and benefits – from the perspective of those on the front lines of projects – that arise through modes of engagement can nuance our thinking about the ethics of engagement with key populations living in impoverished and rights-constrained settings such as Malawi.

'Victims of research'

In January 2013, we (CB and GT) were discussing the state of HIV research within Malawi's sexual minorities populations. Jokingly, GT, the executive director of Centre for the Development of People (CEDEP), Malawi's major LGBTI-rights organization, suggested that men who have sex with men (MSM) have become 'victims of research.' Rising interest in the epidemiological significance of 'key populations' like MSM in countries where homosexuality is illegal or stigmatized has drawn increased funding for populations previously left out of official HIV responses (Parker et al., 1998). In recent years, key populations (KPs), including LGBTI persons, have been prioritized in the global AIDS response, and the Global Fund emphasis on engaging KPs 'at every stage of the funding cycle' has proven to be an avenue for policy change (Global Fund, 2016, 2017). The Global Fund, which, in 2015, disbursed to Malawi the largest allocation of funds to any country or organization ever, places KPs at the core of their global strategy and their investment in these populations has given organizations such as CEDEP leverage in overcoming national barriers, namely homophobia, to service delivery and interventions. In fact, the influx of resources for organizations working with MSM, in particular, has produced a competitive ethos where organizations 'crowd into the KP space' to get a 'piece of the pie.'[1]

In terming MSM 'victims of research,' GT draws attention to how research and other activities that engage MSM carry risks, benefits and unintended consequences. For MSM who joined a cross-sectional HIV study implemented by CEDEP and funded by a US university in 2011–2012, for example, the general sense, implied by non-therapeutic research, that all Malawian MSM's life circumstances in the future might improve because of the findings was balanced against the risk of being found out or associated with a 'gay' project. Meanwhile, in 2017, a cadre of 176 LGBTI peer-educators on the front lines of CEDEP projects balance the benefits of a small monthly stipend and gratification they receive as volunteers against fears that clients might blackmail them by threatening to expose their sexual identity, police might harass them, or that they might be beaten up.[2] Further, as MSM may begin to feel 'over-researched' amid funding infrastructures centered on reducing HIV transmission between men (McKay, 2016), other sexual minorities – e.g. lesbian-identified individuals – have received less attention and fewer resources amid the dominant 'HIV-lens' (cf. Miller, 2016).

CEDEP is the primary and longest running organization working with LGBTI persons in Malawi; it is fully donor funded and invested in 'evidence-based advocacy' toward improving quality of life for Malawi's LGBTI citizens. In recent years, through partnerships with foreign universities and donors, CEDEP has conducted research studies on HIV prevalence, socio-behavioral characteristics and population size of MSM and provided basic community level services, including peer education, distribution of safe sex materials (such as condoms and lubricants), and referrals to friendly health service providers. Alongside this work, CEDEP implements education and advocacy programming, including, for example, training traditional leaders, law enforcers, lawyers, and journalists in LGBTI issues, and lobbying for inclusion of safer sex commodities in Malawi's essential drugs list. CEDEP's work in these arenas, and staff salaries and organizational operational costs, are primarily project-based, meaning funds and resources may be ample at one point and then scarce at another: thus, a large portion of the everyday work of NGO is authoring grant proposals or concept notes for future funding.

It is from within this thicket of advocacy and research work in Malawi that we share our thoughts on community engagement; the next section elaborates the nature of our work with CEDEP, respectively. Before presenting empirical insights drawn from our experiences within NGO spaces, we broaden some of the 'givens' associated with terminologies underlying the interests of this special issue. First, we argue for a more capacious definition of research that includes NGO project-based activities that exceed systematic data collection. Second, we invite readers to imagine community engagement not merely as strategy for improving ethics or enhancing research but as ambivalent process of building trust and suspicion and bringing benefits and harms to communities, many of which are invisible if we think only within normative bounded frames for engagement and ethics. We analyze vignettes drawn from everyday NGO spaces, focusing on how LGBTI volunteer peer educators learn to navigate an economy of harms, or network of social relations and transactions that are simultaneously risky and potentially profitable. We conclude by calling for more empirical attention to *engagement on the ground,* to the everyday relations and transactions that transpire in transnational spaces, rather than to *engagement on paper,* centered on evaluating community engagement's efficacy through indicators, metrics, and measuring.

Methods and context

CEDEP was established over ten years ago to address the needs and challenges of sexual minority and other vulnerable groups in Malawi, particularly regarding human rights, health and social development. When Steven Monjeza and 'Auntie Tiwo' – a male and a transwoman, respectively – engaged in a traditional engagement ceremony (*chinkhoswe*) in 2009, they were tried for unnatural offenses under a colonial era anti-sodomy code, and CEDEP provided them with legal and other support, boosting its organizational profile (Biruk, 2014; Chanika, Lwanda, & Muula, 2013). Locally, CEDEP faces accusations in national media and political rhetoric that it recruits young people to a gay lifestyle, and has witnessed the arrest of its human rights defenders, vandalism of their offices, and backlash against staff. Other human rights organizations in Malawi are hesitant to publicly proclaim support for LGBTI rights and many fear aligning with CEDEP amid fears of political reprisal (Currier, 2015).

This paper is co-produced by Gift (GT), Malawian executive director of [NGO], and Crystal (CB), an American anthropologist. We first met in 2008 at a research dissemination meeting in Malawi sponsored by the National AIDS Commission (NAC). The meeting developed into a collaboration, which has seen GT and CB working together on grant writing, advocacy projects, authoring short essays for public audiences (Biruk & Trapence, 2017), and compiling a book of life stories of gender non-conforming individuals (Xaba & Biruk, 2016). CB and GT are currently undertaking an ethnographic history of LGBTI activism and knowledge production, and CEDEP.

As an anthropologist (CB) and activist director of an NGO (GT), we hold different positions in a larger global health-human rights apparatus, nonetheless undergirded by a common investment in improving conditions for LGBTI Malawians. CB has been working in Malawi since 2005, and began spending time in earnest with CEDEP in 2013, shadowing NGO staff and peer educators, assisting CEDEP with taking minutes at meetings and policy forums, with proposals and reports, and co-leading safer sex trainings, etc. CB has spent over one year on the ground with CEDEP as a volunteer and observant participant in everyday activities between 2013 and 2017. GT, meanwhile, oversees CEDEP's everyday operations and spends much time mediating relationships with foreign donors and researchers, and engages in administrative work associated with managing and overseeing CEDEP's many projects. He also devotes much time to advocacy work, fielding questions and interviews from media within and outside of Malawi and heads efforts to hold government accountable for issues that extend outside the sexual minorities box (i.e. human rights more generally, good governance, etc). Through this work, we have had many conversations about some of the contradictions of North–South collaborations, and about the risks faced by peer educators and other minor actors whose activities are instrumental to carrying out research and intervention, but whose labor often goes under or uncompensated. In 2013, we began formulating this paper, which draws on ethnographic examples and interviews collected by CB and on GT's first-hand experience with CEDEP.

As an academic and an activist, respectively, our lenses and language for analyzing the social phenomena described in this paper differ. In addition, our writing habits take different forms. Whereas GT often writes quickly, authoring press releases, abstracts, concept notes, and shooting off emails to donors, CB, as an academic anthropologist, engages in what Adams, Burke, and Whitmarsh (2014) call 'slow research,' and has the privilege of time to take pause, and to pay attention to social interactions in a meta-way. While on the ground with CEDEP, CB is often charged with taking comprehensive notes on workshops, trainings, and everyday office life that will later be converted into monitoring and evaluation data or donor reports; some examples in this paper are reconstructed from such notes that, in many cases, served also as 'fieldnotes.' Given the different temporalities and urgencies of our respective professions, this paper was primarily written by CB, but much of the material is drawn from fieldnotes recording conversations between GT and CB. We also had Skype meetings to discuss vignettes and examples in the paper, and when we were together in Malawi in 2017, we co-authored and fine-tuned sections of the paper.

Beyond research: unsettling 'engagement' in an economy of harms

'Community engagement' is a framework or model meant to make global health research more ethical, and to address North–South power inequalities between researchers and the researched. While the term is capacious and multiply defined, it has been streamlined into ethics guidance documents, and generally implies working collaboratively with groups of people to improve relevance or ethical conduct of research activities. Engagement foregrounds interactive relationships between communities and research entities; scholars and practitioners who evaluate community engagement are invested in ensuring these relationships are, for example, 'authentic,' 'inclusive,' 'meaningful,' and 'respectful.' Engagement centers dialogue and listening between research teams and research participants, and aims to shift away from a narrow focus on ethics grounded in the consenting individual and toward an ethics that respects the interests of a collective or community (Cyril, Smith, Possamai-Inesedy, & Renzaho, 2015; Holzer, Ellis, & Merritt, 2014; MacQueen et al., 2015; Tindana et al., 2011).

While many of these authors are concerned with the importance of defining what is meant by 'community,' few have explicitly reflected on what it means to engage, even if they suggest the importance of building bridges, relationships, and dialogue across the researcher/researched divide. Existing literature focuses primarily on engagement as something that happens between 'researchers' and 'research participants' and a strategy or goal to be achieved, although King et al. (2014, p. 2) helpfully draw attention to the larger human infrastructure that conducting research relies on. Building on their interest in this 'web of relationships between researchers and the stakeholder community – the unique collection of diverse stakeholders who have interests in the conduct and/or outcomes of a given research project,' this paper expands the frame for thinking about the ethics of engagement beyond researchers and research communities.

CEDEP is an ideal site from which to undertake this expansion, because, while it is implementing some projects explicitly named as 'research,' much of its work falls outside traditional definitions of the term. NGOs such as CEDEP are bridges or brokers between researchers and the researched, or donors and beneficiaries. Research implies the systematic collection of data toward answering a research question, the analysis of that data, and their presentation in published papers. While CEDEP has undertaken such efforts in collaboration with foreign researchers, the bulk of its everyday activity does not match the linear trajectory from chaos to order sketched here. However, CEDEP produces an avalanche of paperwork – monitoring and evaluation forms, donor reports, reports of human rights violations, peer educators' encounter reports, per diem sheets collected at NGO trainings, and so on. Much of this paperwork, symptom of what Davis, Kingsbury, and Merry (2015) call 'governance by indicators' amid an NGO boom in Africa qualifies as 'grey literature;' unlike the products of research proper, it never enters formal circuits of publication and circulation.

Yet, the human infrastructure necessary to collect and collate this information is immense, and implementing any project, whether research or otherwise, necessitates engagement, or building trust and relationships between those who are on the front lines (peer educators, for example), and NGO staff, donors, or members of the LGBTI-identified community. Each of these interfaces, many of which exceed the researcher/researched binary, is characterized by potential for mistrust and suspicion, by transactions caught up in moral economies, and by power relationships that impinge on the outcomes of a given project. Attention to these interfaces sheds useful light on the questions of interest to this special issue.

While funds for research, advocacy, or other programming in NGO spaces originate in wealthy countries, implementation of projects, trainings, or data collection relies on Malawians who have the local knowledge, social networks, and cultural capital to make a project run smoothly. These forms of labor undertaken in the 'field' are often overlooked amid data-driven and donor-driven agendas that collect evidence in the quickest possible fashion and rely on metrics that claim to measure success, but rarely center the stories and experiences of those most vulnerable in the apparatus. Anthropologists and others have shown how the rosy rhetoric of collaboration and participation – common to research and other programming – masks asymmetries and power relationships (Brown, 2015; Crane, 2010; Gerrets, 2015; Kenworthy, 2014; Mercer, 2003). In addition to their contributions to knowledge production being undervalued, peer educators and staff members associated with CEDEP – nationally known for its work with LGBTI persons and other stigmatized groups – are mocked, attacked, or presumed to be gay amid widespread homophobia. Peer educators are entangled in what we term an economy of harms, whereby they seek potential compensation, community, or social mobility even as they subject themselves to risks through affiliation with 'gay' projects. In what follows, we trace how LGBTI people are drawn into this network of social relations that hinges on transactions and obligations that are simultaneously risky and potentially profitable. We present a series of vignettes to show how the ethics of engaging key populations must be responsive not just to narrow project-based parameters undergirded by ethical review, but also to LGBTI Malawians' overlapping social, economic, and political worlds.

Less visible risks in the economy of harms

Following critiques of outsider-led health research in the global South, community engagement is central to responsible knowledge production in impoverished settings and particularly with key populations, and may be a means to recuperate damaged relationships or mistrust between communities and researchers (Trapence et al., 2012; African Key Populations Expert Group, 2014; Molyneux et al., 2016). Rightfully so, research proposals focusing on key populations in Africa – defined as at increased risk for HIV and characterized by social exclusion and stigma – face strict scrutiny when they undergo ethical review by foreign and local institutional review boards (IRBs), who affirm the importance of meaningful contributions from communities affected by research. In its emphasis on showing respect and involving people in design and implementation of research or other projects, community engagement might contribute to the ethical quality of research carried out among vulnerable populations by minimizing harms, though some have shown how such engagement may also *cause* harm (King et al., 2014; Lorway et al., 2014; Molyneux et al., 2016).

However, discussions of avoiding harm, both in cornerstone ethical documents and in secondary literature, tend to: (1) Privilege a definition of harm centered on observable bodily or mental suffering – individual or collective – resulting from research participation; (2) Dominantly focus on biomedical research or clinical trials (Hoeyer & Hogle, 2014; Ndebele, Mfutso-Bengo, & Mduluza, 2008; Petryna, 2005; Wendland, 2008). This bias imbues 'harm' with normative form as visible, adverse bodily/health-centered event (though some authors have expanded this frame to address the social value of research in biomedical settings, see Fairhead, Leach, & Small, 2006 and Zvonareva & Akrong, 2015). We broaden such definitions in two ways. First, we show how harm can result simply from raising expectations or generating feelings of obligation among those who belong to a community of interest. Second, we show that dominant approaches to mitigating harm, such as community engagement, rely on the presumption that 'research' is a bounded activity to be governed, rather than a situated practice that stretches across multiple worlds participants navigate.

A focus on formal aspects of engagement (as GT terms it, 'engagement on paper') – community advisory boards, engagement as ethical practice, and engagement as enhancement of science – means few have explored in detail the behind-the-scenes effects and influence of engagement (and accompanying 'non-obvious risks') on communities (King et al., 2014). Attention to lesser known risks as they arise within mundane spaces and activities common to NGO worlds can enhance researchers' ability to imagine harm and risk in more nuanced ways that are attentive to the social dynamics and transactions that constitute everyday social worlds, and inevitably affect research carried out with LGBTI persons. The next section will describe how the structure of CEDEP's peer education program institutionalizes patron/client relationships between CEDEP and peer educators, with implications for how the latter morally evaluate and come to expect things from CEDEP.

Voluntary labor in the economy of harms

On many weekdays, two or three young people sit in the chairs in CEDEP's office.[3] They socialize among themselves, waiting to drop off forms they use to document the numbers of LGBTI-persons they reach with condoms, lubricants, and safer sex messages. Most days, these peer educators are 'in the field,' engaging LGBTI-persons they meet through personal connections. They distribute educational materials and condoms and lubricants, lead trainings, recruit LGBTI persons for research studies or workshops, collect data, provide referrals to LGBTI-friendly health service providers, and report human rights violations to CEDEP. Peer educators receive a small stipend each month to incentivize their voluntary labor; determining how to balance the voluntary nature of peer education activities with the need to keep peer educators motivated is a dilemma for CEDEP, GT notes. In recent years, thanks to CEDEP's insistence that peer educators should receive more money for their work (and their advocacy for larger budget lines in grants that mobilize peer educators), the stipend has increased (from about 15 USD per month in 2014 to about 32 dollars per month in 2017). In addition, CEDEP now provides a stipend of around 100 dollars per month to a few supervisors who oversee and coordinate peer educator teams. Peer educators, though they are at the lowest echelon of funding and organizational infrastructure, are crucial to the success of NGO programs. Yet, due to donor delays, they often gripe that they are not paid their small monthly stipends on time. Peer educators tend to blame CEDEP for these delays, unaware of the complicated entanglements and relationships through which funds and other benefits reach the lower echelons of organizational infrastructure.

Peer educators are deemed skilled and compassionate advocates, and charged with being upstand-ing, mature, and professional. They hold an MSCE certificate[4] and understand English and at least one local language (commonly, Chewa, Yao, Tumbuka). As LGBTI individuals from the 'same group' as their clients, they are assumed to be able to 'empathize and understand the emotions, thoughts, feelings, language of the participants, and therefore, relate better.'

Only if they properly document the number and form of their encounters into tables are peer edu-cators given monetary incentives for their work. As a memorandum of understanding (MOU) the peer educators sign when they begin volunteering states, incentives 'depend on the resources available' at any given time and may dry up if project contracts end, indicating the coming and going of institu-tional partners and pointing to the fluctuating whims of donors. Peer educators' behavior in the field is guided by a list of ethical standards in the MOU, including maintaining confidentiality, preserving boundaries between peer educators and clients, and avoiding abuse of power in the peer educator/client relationship. Such guidelines become murky when they enter the contexts in which LGBTI-persons' cultural, social, and sexual lives unfold. Due to the small and tightly knit nature of networks, for example, it might be difficult for peer educators to maintain clear distinctions between the 'personal' and the 'professional,' between a lover and a client. As one peer educator put it in a conversation with CB, 'We all stick together.'

In being named 'volunteers,' peer educators' work is recognized as altruistic rather than as labor (Maes, 2017; Prince & Brown, 2016; Sambakunsi, Kumwenda, Choko, Corbett, & Desmond, 2015). Peer educators carry out a variety of tasks on the frontlines of NGO projects, many of which produce 'data' (such as number of clients reached or condoms distributed as filled in to reporting forms) even if it is collected outside traditional research projects. CEDEP's PE model has proven a great asset for recruiting and enrolling peers in research studies, especially in a country where LGBTI persons remain 'underground.' Whereas significant effort is put into protecting confidentiality and ensuring high ethical standards are met when thinking about marginalized or vulnerable research participants or target populations, less is invested in considering ethical issues inherent in relying on peer educator volunteers who implement projects in the field. Although peer educators are touted for 'maintaining high retention and increasing the knowledge of and access to HIV information and services for underserved MSM' in donor reports, the everyday challenges they face are largely invisible to those who aim to create ethical guidelines that pro-tect vulnerable populations from harms that might accrue in the course of research and interventions.

For example, the visibility of peer educators in Malawi and their association with a 'gay organiza-tion' and with known or assumed gays means they may feel threatened or fearful navigating a society unfriendly to those known or presumed to be gay. PEs suggested that they were called 'all kinds of [mean] names,' and reported being blackmailed, for example, upon meeting a new client who threat-ened to 'expose' the peer educator to the community. Peer educators must meet quotas, documented on a report sheet, of distributing materials and interacting with clients in order to receive their monthly stipends; this is sometimes difficult when peers refuse to sign attendance sheets or fear giving their real name amid threats of homophobic violence or blackmail. CEDEP staff members have been arrested for carrying HIV-prevention materials targeting MSM, viewed by law enforcement as 'pornography;' this puts peer educators, who regularly carry condoms and MSM-targeted information in backpacks provided to them by CEDEP, likewise at risk. Fear of exposure and threats against LGBTI-persons in a homophobic context means some PEs accuse CEDEP of 'remain[ing] quiet' in the face of their suffering. They suggested that CEDEP should take responsibility to protect them, because being associated with CEDEP puts them at risk of attacks. These and other examples CB has documented since 2013 – such as LGBTI clients arguing they should be paid because CEDEP 'wouldn't exist without us [LGBTI persons]' – illustrate the transactional nature of trust. Whereas trust is often cast as an ideal endpoint or achievement in community engagement literature, empirical observation within NGO spaces indicates that even as CEDEP provides a welcome safe space and even, in their own words, a 'family' for LGBTI persons, they level criticisms and accusations against CEDEP in the tenor of patron/client relations. CEDEP, on its part, would wish to provide more such protections to its clients, to furnish them with paying jobs, or build a safe house for LGBTI-persons, but absence of funding for such endeavors amid the dominant HIV-lens has stalled these plans. 'Engaging' LGBTI persons – that is involving them in meaningful ways in implementing projects on the ground – produces new kinds of social relations, affects, and tensions within an organization.

While peer educators accuse CEDEP of not offering them enough 'protection' in the field, donor-derived funding structures for such projects often do not devote sufficient budget lines to protections that could improve their security. For example, when CEDEP experienced immense pressure from one donor to collect timely data about key populations, the donor was reluctant to supply staff with vehicles. As GT suggests, one of the largest challenges in working with foreign partners is their failure to recognize significant mobility challenges in a country like Malawi with poor roads and long distances between field sites. CEDEP now has offices across Malawi, and funders often call for frequent monitoring of project activities at all sites. In the absence of enough vehicles, such work is difficult. Vehicles would not only make targets and quotas for data collection more easily achieved but also provide security against violence and attacks peer educators experience on foot. One peer educator said he feels like a 'marked man' as a regular at workshops on gay issues, and is regularly beaten as he walks along the main path near the market.

While ethical guidelines for compensation for *participation* [i.e. surrendering data to research projects via survey responses or blood tests] in clinical trials or research studies are clearly spelled out, there is less clarity around how or whether to best compensate individuals who literally make a project work, such as peer educators: this, too, is a form of participation in projects (cf. Hunter & Ross, 2013). Volunteering, the dominant rhetoric goes, should be preserved as an altruistic gift offered toward the good of one's larger community, rather than become a paid job. A recent 'Lessons Learned' consultant's report about CEDEP's peer education program, for example, suggested that CEDEP should recruit peer educators who are committed to the project and 'not just…there for the money' (Bandawe, 2014, p. 13). Such findings affirm connotations of altruism and generosity carried by the term 'volunteer,' even as they obscure the fact that volunteers rely on the 'salary' they collect for doing what they see as a job. Amid desires for more pay and protections, however, peer educators were committed to their work helping fellow LGBTI persons.

Receiving small stipends – and per diems here and there for attending workshops and trainings – becomes a survival strategy amid rampant joblessness in one of the poorest countries in the world. LGBTI-identified Malawians, it might be said, broker their socially unsavory sexual identities to gain access to potential benefits. CEDEP – and the safer space it provides to those not welcome in church or family arrangements – becomes a key patron in LGBTI-persons' constellation of social relations. NGO bureaucracies, then, become entwined with and reliant on patron-client relations, where cash stipends, transport allowances, equipment (such as the backpacks and binders distributed to peer educators), meals, and airtime are immediate benefits desired by peer educators who enact a kind of 'therapeutic clientship' (Whyte 2014, p. 58). CEDEP and its cadre of peer educators engage in transactions that strengthen bonds between them, but also elevate expectations of continued support.

While LGBTI persons in Malawi appreciate the trainings, information, health services, condoms, and lubricants they gain access to through engagement with CEDEP, their most acutely felt need is economic support, loans, or jobs. The items they receive from CEDEP stoke their hopes, and call upon them to become certain kinds of people so they might benefit from the CEDEP's largesse in the future.

'Volunteering' is motivated and informed by economic desires and an imagined better future (Maes, 2017). By valorizing an ideal type volunteer who eschews greed and self-interest, donors, researchers, and consultants, however, delegitimate peer educators' claims that they deserve more, should be properly paid, or at least receive their stipends on time. As GT points out, projects designed through an 'HIV lens' – centered on testing, treatment and prevention – largely fail to address the other, sometimes more pressing challenges, faced by peer educators and their clients: poverty and lack of vocational skills, for example. The HIV-lens relies on assumptions that people are 'patients' or 'research subjects,' which necessarily limits our ability to imagine or envision harms that befall peer educators, for example, outside of the bounded spaces and times associated with research or hospitals. Further, when research projects are implemented in collaboration with organizations such as CEDEP, the patron/client relationships that predate the research to be undertaken must be accounted for. Research does not begin with a proposal to be implemented; in drawing on pre-existing human infrastructures such as the one assembled by an NGO, it instead becomes another patron in the economy of harms that actors like peer educators navigate.

Benefits in the economy of harms

Community engagement is framed in the literature as a useful strategy for improving ethical outcomes of research, including fair distribution of burdens and benefits. In the context of research projects, benefits are usually framed as after-the-fact results of research that might come to a community in the future or as related to the therapeutic value of participation (for example, receiving health care or medicines). However, from our vantage point within an NGO that implements diverse kinds of projects, research and otherwise, this section shows that 'benefits' can encompass less visible, even seemingly insignificant, resources transacted in the course of a project's unfolding. Yet, harms are perpetually lurking beneath such benefits. This section will also briefly discuss conspiracy theories circulating within CEDEP – that sometimes came 'true' – regarding its infiltration by 'fake gays' and others who seek to expose or blackmail 'real gays,' or steal resources meant for the latter.

A major role of peer educators is to distribute safer sex materials and information to LGBTI persons in the field. Shortages of materials were a common occurrence in 2014, which reduced the credibility of peer educators and decreased interest of clients in continued engagement with CEDEP. In 2014, for example, lubricants were available only irregularly for MSM (Arreola, Hebert, Makofane, Beck, & Ayala, 2012; Bandawe, 2015) and part of CEDEP's advocacy work that year was pushing for inclusion of condom-compatible water-based lubricants in the essential medicines supply list, which would make the Ministry of Health responsible for making this commodity accessible. As noted in a policy paper, lubricants are associated with men who have sex with men (MSM), making those who would ask for them in a pharmacy (where they carry a high price) feel ashamed to do so. Health care providers and government officials alike suggested that distributing lubricants would encourage homosexuality in Malawi, where laws named same sex relations as illegal.[5]

Whereas we tend to think of the 'benefits' of participating in research or other projects far into the future (health services, access to medicines, policy change, etc), on the ground, many people participate in order to receive immediate benefits and expect some payoff for time, energy or information they give up (Reynolds, Cousins, Newell, & Imrie, 2013, p. 122). In considering the implications and consequences of involving local people in projects, we should take note of the less visible benefits, beyond medicines or health care, that people come to value, desire, and stake claims on. In this case, MSM who learn about and access condoms and lubricants via peer educators expect these objects as new and normative features of their sex lives, perhaps symbolic of sexual modernity (Nguyen, 2005). Safer sex workshops that educate participants about lubricants do not just fulfill a need, but produce one. In the economy of harms, newly valuable and desired items such as lubricants are benefits that carried, in 2014, the risk of exposure in trying to access them from private pharmacies, and the harm of the absent presence of a safer sex commodity MSM elsewhere take for granted (In 2017, lubricants are now widely accessible through CEDEP).

LGBTI persons' exposure to trainings, workshops, and new knowledge may prompt them to articulate demands for more benefits, including human rights. Following LGBTI health trainings in 2013, for example, lesbian-identified workshop participants took up the language of human rights: 'The government should be providing us with those [dental] dams. It is our human right to have them.' The absence of lubricants and dental dams at the time – even as they are 'present' in template-training materials, discussions, and workshops as objects of knowledge and standards for LGBTI safe sex – illustrates how NGO forums and spaces cultivate new desires and how immediate benefits (even in the form of tiny commodities like dental dams or lubricants) are discussed, desired, and become sites of claimsmaking, as in the articulation of dams as human rights or health entitlements. LGBTI-identified Malawians' engagement in research and other projects (such as trainings and workshops) cultivates new expectations and demands, whether for lubricants, social support, higher stipends or per diems, or even jobs.

In the case of peer educators who view volunteering as a form of labor and incentives as a salary (Folayan, Haire, Harrison, Fatusi, & Brown, 2014), the influx of resources into NGOs provides opportunities for people who are jobless and struggling to make ends meet in one of the poorest countries in the world. Such resources (transport allowances, meals, per diems, e.g.) can become sites of friction and debate on the ground. For example, when CEDEP staff hold workshops, they often are held to quotas and guidelines from funding organizations. A training might be targeted at 15 gay men and 10 lesbians and five transgender individuals. Peer educators and staff members are responsible for sourcing these individuals (parsed by sexual orientation) and, in line with global health and human rights audit culture rooted in quantifying the number of beneficiaries reached by such trainings, having them sign a document attesting their attendance and receipt of per diems.

Seats at workshops were coveted because they carry per diems, include lunch, cookies, sodas, and bottled water, and provide a site to socialize. The limited distribution of these much desired 'benefits' – deemed unjust by those who were excluded – created jealousies and tensions (See AmFAR, 2011 for a discussion of T-shirts, food, and other small incentives as major motivation for participation in a study on pre-exposure prophylaxis (PrEP) in MSM in Cape Town).

Among themselves, Malawian LGBTI people also discussed 'fake gays,' individuals who were pretending: (1) To be gay; or (2) To be allies to LGBTI, claiming that they were 'infiltrating our space.' CEDEP had to arbitrate the authenticity of accused fake gays' sexual orientations when trusted peer educators informed staff members that some among them were attending workshops merely to earn per diems. Sussing out someone's sexual orientation upon meeting them is an odd, if not impossible task, but demonstrates the very real fear that fake gays might embed themselves to feed information to those in Malawi who oppose the 'gay agenda' or, at the very least, steal benefits meant for 'real gays.'

When we view workshops (and incentives they carry) as immediate benefits valued by populations being engaged, we see how and why people might conspire to infiltrate them. At a training held in June 2014 for 20 health service providers (HSPs) at a district hospital, MSM sat alongside non-LGBTI identified HSPs such as doctors, nurses, and other intake staff. Attendees to the workshop, funded by a Dutch NGO and a British organization, received a per diem, lodging and meals. Part of the workshop's objective was to put a face to the stigmatized category 'MSM' and to allow HSPs to overcome their fears about interacting with MSM. The MSM present were suspicious of a male HSP at the training, whom they accused of being homophobic, of sitting in on the training merely to claim his money; they claimed he would go back to the hospital and 'out' them. This accusation – that 'he [was] not doing it for the right reasons' – embeds numerous dynamics that underlie 'economies of harm' in NGO worlds in Malawi: Not only would this man potentially put MSM at risk, but he was taking money away from a deserving person who could have come instead. Further, the idea that he could go back to his workplace and out the MSM he now knew by sight points to the importance of thinking about the ethics of engagement through a diachronic and socially embedded, rather than a presentist and impersonal lens. While training HSPs is part of an ethical project to reduce homophobia and improve health care for MSM, it unexpectedly might, at least in their view, subject them to *more harm*.

Conclusion

We have illustrated that 'engagement' can produce, even as it aims to reconcile, expectations between participants and projects. Attention to small transactions – of lubricants, information, per diems, stipends, and so on – and cycles of obligation that arise through engagement illustrates some of the less visible 'harms' beyond those related to health or the body that arise from this social form. Within donor-constrained projects, LGBTI Malawians are expected to participate in a wide variety of research, education, and advocacy projects altruistically or toward the larger good of their community. Engagement is widely perceived to be a corrective to outsider-driven research agendas and projects, but it is important to note that it carries significant risks and produces new kinds of obligation, social relations, and expectations. LGBTI persons in Malawi are conscious of how their engagements with various projects inherently subject them to harms (beyond those imagined by ethics committees or project visions), and of the imbalance they experience between risks and benefits within and outside the context of formal research. CEDEP, for example, has become a key patron in peer educators' network of support.

Operating ambivalently within an 'economy of harms', LGBTI-identified peer educators invite us to not only call for more or better engagement, but to critically consider the unpredictable consequences and social relations that arise in infrastructures of engagement. They help us see how publics are enacted in concert with research and interventions; the 'community' does not pre-exist such projects, nor is it comprised only of those most obviously 'engaged' under the rubric of community engagement frameworks, primarily research participants or target populations (Montgomery & Pool, 2017). Amid calls to implement 'standard and reliable measures' to gauge whether engagement leads to enhanced ethical outcomes, we suggest it is more pressing to learn from the everyday, largely invisible, struggles of those on the front lines of projects, such as peer educators. Our long-term observations working on the ground and in CEDEP's offices, captured some of the less visible harms (and benefits) that arise in relations and transactions that may fall outside the bounded definition of 'research', but nonetheless affect such undertakings. We advocate for attention to the everyday empirical realities into which all projects enter: while research is conducted under time constraints and data-driven, small shifts in our attention – toward mundane, for example, rather than adverse events – might come about through the kind of 'slowing down' of global health research advocated by Adams et al. (2014). Learning from those on the frontlines of projects, in addition to those cast as research participants, can teach us that even as community engagement builds social networks, it also generates an economy of harms that takes shape amid circuits of resource distribution in Africa.

Nyambedha (2008, p. 775), an ethnographer of global health, proposes that we define 'harm' broadly to include raising research subjects' expectations without addressing them. Plans for engagement must account for the complex social, political, and economic contexts that inform LGBTI persons' assessments and felt experiences of engagement as risky, if potentially profitable, business. Ethics and engagement are concepts easily articulated on paper, but only rarely is close attention paid to the ad hoc and informal aspects of engagement on the ground. In an era of global health increasingly dominated by a focus on data, targets and metrics that measure ostensibly successful outcomes, we can too easily lose sight of the faces behind the data points – not just research participants or clients, but also those who recruit them. As GT points out, implementing organizations like CEDEP are too often on the 'receiving end' of research projects that come to them whole cloth and pre-packaged, also with pre-defined notions of harm and benefits conceived from a top-down perspective. Finally, we suggest that NGOs are a fitting and overlooked site from which to consider questions around the everyday politics and practices of engagement. First, they are important partners for research projects or key entry points into hidden or underground communities such as MSM. Second, NGOs like CEDEP are key patrons for LGBTI persons and close attention to the nature of obligations, expectations and circulation of resources in NGO spaces can help us meaningfully attend to socio-material expectations that pre-exist or exceed research.

Notes

1. Fieldnotes, meeting on global fund grant, NGO offices, June 5, 2017.
2. In the wake of such incidents, CEDEP provides peer educators with safety and security trainings, and established a toll-free help line where LGBTI can report violent incidents. CEDEP has also strengthened connections between police victim units and LGBTI persons.
3. All peer educators identify as MSM or transwomen. While CEDEP wishes to implement more extensive programming for lesbian- and transmale identified individuals, donors' disproportionate focus on mitigating HIV transmission has, in GT's words, 'left lesbians [and transmen] in the cold.'
4. Malawi Certificate of Education Examination, indicating a person has passed the national exam at the end of secondary school.
5. In July 2016, the Tanzanian government banned lubricants in an effort to 'curb homosexuality' ('Tanzania bans lubricant,' July 23, 2016).

Disclosure statement

No potential conflict of interest was reported by the authors.

Funding

This work was supported by Oberlin College Powers Grants and The Wenner-Gren Foundation [grant number 9179].

References

Adams, V., Burke, N., & Whitmarsh, I. (2014). Slow research: Thoughts for a movement in global health. *Medical Anthropology, 33*(3), 179–197.

African Key Populations Expert Group. (2014). *Model regional strategic framework on HIV for key populations in Africa*. UNDP.

AmFAR. 2011. *Best practices guidance in conducting HIV research with gay, bisexual and other MSM in rights-constrained environments*. New York, NY: AmFAR.

Arreola, S., Hebert, P., Makofane, K., Beck, J., & Ayala, G. 2012. *Access to HIV prevention and treatment for MSM: Findings from the 2012 GMHR study*. Oakland, CA: The Global Forum on MSM & HIV (MSMGF).

Bandawe, C. (2014). *Lessons learned from the [NGO] peer educators programme*. Unpublished manuscript.

Bandawe, C. (2015). *A survey on alternative sexual reproductive health services available for LGBTIQ in 3 districts of Malawi*. Lilongwe: CHRR + UFBR.

Biruk, C. (2014). 'Aid for gays': The moral and the material in 'African homophobia' in post-2009 Malawi. *The Journal of Modern African Studies, 52*(3), 447–473.

Biruk, C., & Trapence G. (2017, April 14). Gay for pay in an economy of harms: Reflections from an LGBTI-rights NGO in Malawi. *Anthropology News*.

Brown, H. (2015). Global health partnerships, governance, and sovereign responsibility in western Kenya. *American Ethnologist, 42*(2), 340–355.

Chanika, E., Lwanda, J., & Muula, A. S. (2013). Gender, gays and gain: The sexualized politics of donor aid in Malawi. *Africa Spectrum, 48*(1), 89–105.

Crane, J. (2010). Unequal 'partners': AIDS, academia and the rise of global health. *Behemoth, 3*, 78–97.

Currier, A. (2015). Arrested solidarity: Obstacles to intermovement support for LGBT rights in Malawi. *WSQ, 42*(3&4), 146–163.

Cyril, S., Smith, B. J., Possamai-Inesedy, A., & Renzaho, A. M. N. (2015). Exploring the role of community engagement in improving the health of disadvantaged populations: A systematic review. *Global Health Action, 8*(1), 29842.

Davis, K. E., Kingsbury, B., & Merry, S. E. (2015). Global governance by indicators. In D. Kevin, A. Fisher, B. Kingsbury, & S. E. Merry (Eds.), *Governance by indicators: Global power through quantification* (pp. 3–28). Oxford: Oxford University Press.

England, C. (2016, July 23). Tanzania bans lubricant in bid to 'curb homosexuality'. *The Independent*.

Fairhead, J., Leach, M., & Small, M. (2006). Where techno-science meets poverty: Medical research and the economy of blood in The Gambia, West Africa. *Social Science and Medicine, 63*(4), 1109–1120.

Folayan, M. O., Haire, B., Harrison, A., Fatusi, O., & Brown, B. (2014). Beyond informed consent: Ethical considerations in the design and implementation of sexual and reproductive health research among adolescents. *African Journal of Reproductive Health, 18*(300), 118–126.

Gerrets, R. 2015. International health and the proliferation of 'partnerships': (Un)Intended boost for state institutions in Tanzania? In P. W. Geissler (Ed.), *Para-states and medical science: Making African global health* (pp. 179–206). Durham, NC: Duke University Press.

Global Fund. 2016. Key populations and the global fund: Delivering key results. Amsterdam: Free Space Process.

Global Fund. 2017. Key populations. Retrieved from https://www.theglobalfund.org/en/key-populations/

Hoeyer, K., & Hogle, L. F. (2014). Informed consent: The politics of intent and practice in medical research ethics. *ARA, 43*, 347–362.

Holzer, J. K., Ellis, L., & Merritt, M. W. (2014). Why we need community engagement in medical research. *Journal of Investigative Medicine, 62*(6), 851–855.

Hunter, K., & Ross, E. (2013). Stipend-paid volunteers in South Africa: A euphemism for low-paid work? *Development Southern Africa, 30*(6), 743–759.

Kenworthy, N. (2014). Participation, decentralisation and déjà vu: Remaking democracy in response to AIDS? *Global Public Health, 9*(1-2), 25–42.

King, K. F., Kolopack, P., Merritt, M. W., & Lavery, J. V. (2014). Community engagement and the human infrastructure of global health research. *BMC Medical Ethics, 15*, 84.

Lorway, R., Thompson, L. H., Lazarus, L., du Plessis, E., Pasha, A., Fathima Mary, P., ... Reza-Paul, S. (2014). Going beyond the clinic: Confronting stigma and discrimination among men who have sex with men in Mysore through community based participatory research. *Critical Public Health, 24*(1), 73–87.

MacQueen, K. M., Bhan, A., Frohlich, J., Holzer, J., Sugarman, J., & Ethics Working Group of the HIV Prevention Trials Network. 2015. Evaluating community engagement in global health research: The need for metrics. *BMC Medical Ethics, 16*(44), 1–9.

Maes, K. 2017. *The lives of community health workers: Local labor and global health in Urban Ethiopia.* New York: Routledge.

McKay, T. (2016). From marginal to marginalized: The inclusion of men who have sex with men in global and national AIDS programmes and policy. *Global Public Health, 11*(7–8), 902–922.

Mercer, C. (2003). Performing partnership: Civil society and the illusions of good governance in Tanzania. *Political Geography, 22*, 741–763.

Miller, C. J. (2016). Dying for money: The effects of global health initiatives on NGOs working with gay men and HIV/AIDS in northwest China. *Medical Anthropology Quarterly, 30*(3), 414–430.

Molyneux, S., Sariola, S., Allman, D., Dijkstra, M., Gichuru, E., Graham, S., ... Sanders, E. (2016). Public/community engagement in health research with men who have sex with men in sub-Saharan Africa: challenges and opportunities. *Health Research Policy and Systems, 14*(40), 1–12.

Montgomery, C. M., & Pool, R. (2017). From 'trial community' to 'experimental public': How clinical research shapes public participation. *Critical Public Health, 27*(1), 50–62.

Ndebele, P., Mfutso-Bengo, J., & Mduluza, T. (2008). Compensating clinical trial participants from limited resource settings in internationally sponsored trials. *Malawi Medical Journal, 20*(2), 42–45.

Nguyen, V.-K. (2005). Uses and pleasures: Sexual modernity, HIV/AIDS, and confessional technologies in a West African metropolis. In V. Adams & S. Leigh Pigg (Eds.), *Sex in development: Science, sexuality and morality in global perspective* (pp. 245–268). Durham, NC: Duke University Press.

Nyambedha, E. O. (2008). Ethical dilemmas of social science research on AIDS and orphanhood in Western Kenya. *Social Science & Medicine, 67*, 771–779.

Parker, R., Khan, S., & Aggleton, P. (1998). Conspicuous by their absence? Men who have sex with men (msm) in developing countries: Implications for HIV prevention. *Critical Public Health, 8*(4), 329–346.

Petryna, A. (2005). Ethical variability: Drug development and globalizing clinical trials. *American Ethnologist, 32*(2), 183–197.

Prince, R., & Brown, H. (Eds.) 2016. *Volunteer economies: The politics and ethics of voluntary labour in Africa.* Melton: James Currey.

Reynolds, L., Cousins, T., Newell, M.-L., & Imrie, J. (2013). The social dynamics of consent and refusal in HIV surveillance in rural South Africa. *Social Science & Medicine, 77*, 118–125.

Sambakunsi, R., Kumwenda, M., Choko, A., Corbett, E. L., & Desmond, N. A. (2015). 'Whose failure counts?' A critical reflection on definitions of failure for community health volunteers providing HIV self-testing in a community-based HIV/TB intervention study in urban Malawi. *Anthropology and Medicine, 22*(3), 234–249.

Tindana, P. O., Rozmovits, L., Boulanger, R. F., Bandewar, S. V. S., Aborigo, R. A., Hodgson, A. V. O., ... Lavery, J. V. (2011). Aligning community engagement with traditional authority structures in global health research: A case study from northern Ghana. *American Journal of Public Health, 101*(10), 1857–1867.

Trapence, G., Collins, C., Avrett, S., Carr, R., Sanchez, H., Ayala, G., ... Baral, S. D. (2012). From personal survival to public health: Community leadership by men who have sex with men in the response to HIV. *The Lancet, 101*(10), 1857–1867.

Wendland, C. (2008). Research, therapy, and bioethical hegemony: The controversy over perinatal AZT trials in Africa. *African Studies Review, 51*(3), 1–23.

Whyte, S. R. (Ed.). (2014). *Second chances: Surviving AIDS in Uganda.* Durham, NC: Duke University Press.

Xaba, K. & Biruk, C. (Eds.). (2016). *Proudly Malawian: Life stories of lesbian and gender non-conforming individuals in Malawi.* Johannesburg: MaThoko's Books.

Zvonareva, O., & Akrong, L. (2015). Developing clinical research relationship: Views from within. *Developing World Bioethics, 15*(3), 257–266.

Emerging dynamics of evidence and trust in online user-to-user engagement: the case of 'unproven' stem cell therapies

Saheli Datta ⓘ

ABSTRACT

This article explores the ways in which patients and their families (hereafter referred as 'users') share and evaluate disease-specific evidence via online communities. The aim is to understand what this user engagement in healthcare and knowledge production reveals about society's shifting perceptions of trust in the institutions of 'evidence-based medicine' (EBM) such as regulators, bioethicists and scientists and the implications for EBM. To do this, I use the case of experimental stem cell therapies (eSCTs). ESCTs are commonly labelled in academic literature as 'unproven', a label that frames their lack of conclusive clinical evidence as unsafe, inefficacious and thus unethical when clinically used. Despite this framing, users engage with other users to share and evaluate all available evidence for themselves, including on-going clinical trial and experiential evidence to build trust for and undertake eSCTs. Increasingly, this user engagement with evidence takes place in online communities that range from user-created and user-run *Facebook* pages to user-to-user discussion forums on healthcare provider sites or blogs with little if any provider-input in conversations. In this paper, I draw on a sample of these user conversations to show the complex and unpredictable ways in which what counts as evidence and how trust is built for it are shifting. In so doing, I reflect on the shifting relations between the institutions of EBM and society for greater control over evidence that lies at the heart of the evidentiary basis of public health policies.

Introduction

In 2012 and 2013, two large-scale surveys of healthcare trends in the US (by *Pew Research* and *PricewaterhouseCoopers*) attempted to quantify an emerging trend of online health information seeking among patients and their families; or what I call user-to-user engagement. The *PricewaterhouseCoopers* (2012) survey found that 32% of adults used social media to follow family or friends' experiences of illness and disease. Twenty-nine per cent of adults sought information related to other patients' experiences with their disease and 24% viewed health-related videos or images posted online by patients. This article explores the dynamics of online user-to-user engagement in healthcare and knowledge production in the specific case of experimental stem cell therapies (eSCTs), for which a majority of patients and their families (hereafter referred to as 'users') build trust for eSCTs through online communities. The aim is to help understand society's shifting perceptions of trust in the institutions of 'evidence-based medicine' (EBM), such as regulators, bioethicists, scientists, etc. (hereafter referred as 'providers') and the implications of these shifts for EBM.

Since the 1980s, social scientists have focused increasing attention upon the relations between science and society in the wake of growing mistrust in scientific knowledge and expertise (Leach, Scoones, & Wynne, 2005; Putnam, 1993; Starr, 1982; Wynne, 2006). Critical scholarship challenged the 'deficit model' that informed efforts to engage publics; a model which assumed that mistrust was due to ignorance or a 'deficit' in knowledge rather than critical thinking and the co-existence of other ways of knowing (Wynne, 2006). Partly in response to this critique and to a combination of large-scale citizen mobilisations (e.g. surrounding HIV/AIDS research in the 90s) and growing discursive engagement with 'more traditional ways of knowing medicine' like experiential evidence (Djulbegovic, Guyatt, & Ashcroft, 2009), more participatory models of EBM integrating experiential evidence have since emerged and become widely practiced, particularly in downstream healthcare settings (Charles, Gafni, & Freeman, 2011; Miles & Mezzich, 2011; Tonelli, 2006).

Against this backdrop, the Internet has generated novel possibilities for publics to engage with evidence and medicine. One such example is the emergence of online communities dedicated to sharing and evaluating the credibility of all available disease-specific evidence including scientific and experiential evidence. What do these spaces reveal about the relations between scientific evidence (from basic research and clinical trials), public trust and scientific evidence as a basis for policy? This paper presents societal engagement from *Facebook* pages and discussion forums surrounding the clinical use of eSCTs. These online spaces can be thought of as online communities in which users share and evaluate available evidence to build trust in eSCTs, alongside traditional provider-based sources of trust-building, such as physicians. For instance, disease-specific discussion forums attract users on the basis of shared (disease-specific) interests and helps foster kinship and knowledge sharing (e.g. discussions on *MS Society UK*) (Wright & Street, 2007). Nevertheless, it is important to emphasise that online user–user engagement represents one increasingly relevant perspective, and not the entirety of experiences and views.

What is notable about these communities for our purposes is the absence of input from 'providers'. I will show that, in a context where eSCT users are viewed as ignorant or gullible (Qiu, 2009), these online spaces can be read as productive sites of user empowerment in producing and evaluating evidence for user choice of eSCTs (Andreassen & Trondsen, 2010; Lupton, 2013). By drawing attention to communities that do not actually want to be 'engaged' by providers, this article offers the provocation that the logic of participation and inclusiveness in existing community and public engagement models may not have gone far enough. Through relating user activity in online user-to-user engagement, this article explores *why* and *how* people produce, evaluate and build trust for evidence. As I will show, users do not simply disfavour scientific evidence in favour of experiential evidence, but rather combine these and other sources of evidence in complex and unpredictable ways. This article, therefore, casts online communities as productive epistemic spaces (in the sense of Haas' (2001, p. 11579) epistemic actors with 'agency in politics and policy formation'), which signal a shift in what counts as evidence and how trust is built for this evidence.

Dynamics of user-to-user engagement

Contemporary public engagement is intended to foster dialogue between policymakers and policy takers and to engender mutual trust. However, critical scholarship has suggested that engagement practices have been and continue to be mere tokenistic gestures by providers in line with 'fashion-following' political rhetoric, and thus largely ineffective in rebuilding public trust (Wynne, 2006, p. 217). Wynne, for instance, showed that expert policymakers were instead interested in downstream 'instrumental concerns about impacts … [and how] these can be identified, and represented, adequately by scientific risk assessment' (Wynne, 2006, p. 218).

In particular, in the context of emerging technologies, there is a long history of contestation over the rights of technology end-users, which has intensified in the last decade (for an exhaustive discussion, see Smith, Bossen, & Kanstrup, 2017). Consider for instance the case of AIDS activism in the 1990s, which highlighted this chasm in the understanding of end-users between provider's imagination of a future user and users' lived experiences (Epstein, 1996; Lambert, 2013). Recent scholarship has sought to bridge this chasm with 'user-centred' technology design based on user experiences instead of 'edited render-ings' of the image of the user to suit specific professional or technological uses (Hyysalo & Johnson, 2015; see e.g. 'human-centred design' in Bazzano, Martin, Hicks, Faughnan, & Murphy, 2017).

In policy-making, the enactment of 'Right-to-Try' legislation nationally and across thirty-seven US states since 2014, which allow terminal patients the 'right to try' experimental treatments without seeking prior FDA approval (Brennan, 2017), highlights this increasing focus on technology end-users. Nevertheless, 'Right-to-Try' laws remain at its heart an 'access debate' (Dresser, 2014) even though they highlight tensions between expert and lay interpretations about the adequacy or accuracy of available evidence in private treatment choices (Pear & Kaplan, 2017). Thus, to what extent access based consider-ations in policy like the UK's *Early Access to Medicines Scheme* launched in December 2014 will translate to meaningful considerations of lived experiences in the evidence basis of EBM remains unclear (Facey et al., 2010; Greenhalgh, Snow, Ryan, Rees, & Salisbury, 2015), although the case for a 'compromise policy' integrating experiential evidence in policy-making is emerging (Matthews & Iltis, 2015).

At the same time, as the *PricewaterhouseCoopers* (2012) survey data presented in the introduction suggest, when it comes to disease-specific evidence and treatments, users are increasingly engaging with other users to seek and share lived experiences (hereafter also referred as 'experiential evidence'). Moreover, this engagement is sought and fostered in user-to-user relationships with little or, no recourse to provider-side inputs (Lupton, 2013). To understand these dynamics of evidence and trust in emerg-ing user-to-user engagement, the contestation between scientific and experiential evidence in eSCTs provides an excellent case study.

Experimental stem cell therapies

Except for a handful of SCTs approved for public marketing, most remain experimental (i.e. lacking conclusive evidence of clinical safety and efficacy) and unavailable to the Euro-American public through public healthcare providers like the UK NHS and the US Medicare. However, eSCTs have been and con-tinue to be available in private clinics in the global south (Lau et al., 2008) and increasingly in OECD countries (Berger et al., 2016; Turner & Knoepfler, 2016). Since the early 2000s, media coverage of the immense potential of stem cells as a 'miracle cure' created public demand for eSCTs (Ramesh, 2005). The result was that Euro-American seekers of eSCTs not only started travelling beyond their home countries to access eSCTs but also, in the absence of clinical evidence, started to seek and share experiential evidence to evaluate the benefits of eSCTs for themselves. In turn, providers used the term 'unproven' to describe eSCTs, highlighting public access to them as unsafe and unethical based on their lack of conclusive clinical evidence of efficacy (ISSCR, 2013; Lau et al., 2008; McLean, Stewart, & Kerridge, 2015).

On the one hand, the effect of a negative label like 'unproven' instead of a label like 'experimental' for experimental SCTs is that 'unproven' not only casts eSCT practitioners as charlatans but also frame users as 'gullible' and lacking the capacity to make good health choices (Qiu, 2009) without provider intervention (Master & Resnik, 2011). Thus, the construct of 'unproven' not only assumes a moral high ground that presupposes scientific evidence as the only legitimate way of knowing therapeutic safety and efficacy but also public trust in its legitimacy. In this sense, 'unproven' frames public trust in eSCTs within the boundaries of scientific evidence and delegitimises those stepping beyond those boundaries when considering 'other' forms of evidence like user experiences (ISSCR, 2008).

On the other hand, the agency of eSCT users who 'bypass' warnings by the 'institutions of stem cell science' is increasingly studied (Salter, Zhou, & Datta, 2015, p. 162; see also Chen & Gottweis, 2013; Lupton, 2013), particularly in studies of how users build trust for experiential evidence through online user–user communities (Bharadwaj, 2012,p 312; Foster, 2016; Kallinikos & Tempini, 2014; Rachul, 2011). For *instance*, Petersen, MacGregor, and Munsie (2016) used the lens of the televised experience of Kristy Cruise – an Australian patient who had travelled to Russia to undertake eSCT – to shed light on the increasingly important role of digital media in shaping hope-risk expectations among users. Perhaps more than anything else, Petersen et al. (2016) highlighted the disease-specific communities that form around similar concerns with evidence and which this paper explores to understand why and how these communities engage with each other, and increasingly through online environments (see e.g. Aubusson, 2014 in McLean et al., 2015). Indeed, Sharpe, Di Pietro, Jacob, and Illes' (2016, p. 441) finding that among 'individuals interested in stem cell tourism … internet was the most commonly cited source for information-seeking, … [with most using] stem cell clinic websites [and] social media', emphasises the need to understand the emerging dynamics of online user–user engagement. This paper extends this growing body of work to understand *why* and *how* users 'step-out' beyond the notion of 'unproven' to evaluate for themselves the credibility of both scientific and experiential evidence via online communities; evaluations of *what* 'experiential data' is shared, provide opportunities for future research. This paper also extends the surveys by *Pew Research* (Pew Research-Fox & Duggan, 2013) and *PricewaterhouseCoopers* (2012) by exploring why user-to-user sharing of disease-specific evidence is happening and how it is building trust in certain kinds of evidence. As this form of engagement is increasingly mediated through online communal spaces like *Facebook* and discussion forums, a sample of user-to-user conversations in these spaces are studied to answer these questions.

Method

Sampling and data collection

In this study, I used two search methods to draw a sample of user conversations. First, using the online *Facebook*-page ranking tool *Socialbakers.com* which ranks pages by user visits, I ranked the most user-visited *Facebook* pages using the search term 'stem cell therapies'[1] (referred to in data extracts below as File1). The search returned 61 *Facebook* pages of which eight were chosen after excluding others based on exclusion criteria including fewer than five user-visits or content relating to non-medical applications such as cosmetic surgery. Of the selected eight *Facebook*-pages, four were moderated and run by patients' families, three by eSCT clinics and one by a private medical tourism facilitator. Second, I took a disease-specific approach, focusing on the top three websites on Multiple Sclerosis (MS) (excluding provider websites offering eSCTs) that users see when they Google 'stem cell therapies multiple sclerosis' namely, the *National Multiple Sclerosis Society* (www.facebook.com/nationalmssociety; 358 of 818 posts; 2014–2016), the *MS Society* (www.mssociety.org.uk; 69 of 818 posts; 2011–2012) and *The Niche* (ipscell. com; 141 of 818 posts; 2012–2016) (referred to in extracts below as Files 2, 3 and 4, respectively). MS was chosen based on Berger et al.'s (2016, pp. 160–161) survey of the 'top [30] conditions treated by all clinics and academic centres' worldwide for eSCTs. The final sample had 818 posts and 20 testimonials drawn from eight Facebook pages and three websites between 2011 and 2016.

This dual search method mimicked the search pattern typically employed by users as identified through informal conversations with eSCT-patients at a private clinic in Delhi, India. The logic of the searches was that, while the Facebook search gave users an array of user-created and -run conversations relating to all conversations in SCTs, the disease-specific search provided disease-specific information and conversations on provider-run sites. Moreover, this sample of *Facebook* and discussion forums is appropriate for this research as both platforms allow users to engage with each other over the long term and forge communities (unlike e.g. *Twitter's* event-centric public engagement) and is consistent with Sharpe et al.'s (2016, p. 441) findings of online community engagement trends in eSCTs. Importantly, this search method is emblematic of the ways in which the geographies of these online communities map into the lived experiences of users who travel globally to access eSCTs unavailable at home.

Analysis

The qualitative data analysis software *Atlas-ti* was used to organise thematic coding of the sample. Codes were derived inductively from my thematic analysis and the broad themes that emerged included issues of trust, distrust, betrayal, sense of victimisation, risk awareness and rationalisation, knowledge gain (and its sources) and knowledge sharing.

Ethics and limitations

A key limitation was that the *Google* search (in the disease-specific approach) generated an abundance of data in excess of one million results, from which only the top three sites were studied. This means that other sites could have revealed data important for this research but could not be studied due to human cognitive and time constraints. Another limitation, as with any social-media research, was the possibility of data inaccuracies arising from (a) 'exaggerated views' posted online, (b) differences between online and 'real-world' behaviours enabled by '[user] anonymity' on the internet (Beninger et al., 2014) and (c) distortion by fake user accounts. Large social networks including *Facebook* were already using dedicated staff and various fake-account detection tools like *SybilsRank*[2] as far back as 2012 (Cao, Sirivianos, Yang, & Pregueiro, 2012), although their effectiveness remains questionable. To reduce fake account distortion, the research used participant 'views', which were repeatedly reflected across the web pages/sites (greater '*n*') at different times by different participants. Lastly, this research was limited to English-language content because social media analytics applications like *socialbakers.com* are algorithmically limited to English content. Interestingly, there were no discernible language proficiency issues because a *Google* search conducted from a UK-based IP address (in an English-speaking region) is designed to return English-centric results – which is limiting. However, reconfiguring Google to each linguistic-region of the world was unfeasible. As regards research ethics, informed consent was deemed unnecessary as (a) only material in the public domain were used and (b) usernames were anonymised (blanked) where direct quotes are used or where possible data was presented in aggregate or paraphrased in accordance with anonymity and 'no harm' requirements (Markham & Buchannan, 2012).

Why users step out beyond the boundaries of 'unproven'

Conversations revealed that participants stepped beyond the boundaries of 'unproven' to evaluate the trustworthiness and credibility of evidence. Decisions to do so were tied to distrust in processes, actors and institutions underpinning scientific evidence, especially those perceived to have commercial linkages, but did not extend to distrust in scientific evidence itself. Participants widely believed in the systemic collusion between 'big pharma' (perceived as dishonest) and regulators, in particular, the US Food and Drug Administration (FDA). The belief that the FDA – the 'protector' of public interests – was colluding against them engendered distrust and a sense of betrayal by institutions of scientific evidence perceived to have significant conflicts of public–private interests (File2, File4). Participants viewed themselves as victims of the profit-driven pharmaceutical industry, which, in collusion with regulators, were perceived to profit from the 'sickness industry':

> The FDA is just in the hip pocket of Big Pharma. Too many drugs [have] been put out as safe and later people are dying from them. As adults we should have a little more freedom to make our own health decisions. (File4-January/2012)

> … big pharmaceutical companies won't allow a cure. Too much money to be made keeping people sick. (File2-June/2016)

Prominent recalls of drugs which had been granted market authorisation by leading regulators such as the FDA, despite the clinical evidence on the contrary, was viewed by participants as instances of regulator–industry collusion against public interests. In stem cells, the *Regenex*[3]-v-FDA case – where the US courts' ruling in favour of FDA regulating *autologous* (patient's own) stem cells-like drugs led to state–public contestation (Eisenstein, 2016) – was viewed by participants as evidence of the FDA's collusion with 'big-pharma' to control and thereby profit from the human body. As one participant summarised:

> … FDA is in bed with the Pharmaceutical, they have been for decades. They have approved thousands of 'legal' drugs on the market, which has resulted in millions of deaths around America, through prescription drugs. … to

say stem cells are drugs is a complete and utter nonsense, it is an organ transplant. It has NOTHING to do with FDA or being a drug. In fact the FDA have persistently tried to shut down all stem cell activities as it is threatening their playground of manufacturing hard drugs and keeping people sick, as opposed to treating them once and for all. Wake up people!!! (File4-January/2012)

Until FDA can figure out how to make money on this, people will suffer financially and in health! (File4-December/2013)

The phrase 'FDA' appeared 35 times among 141 posts in response to the 'Top 10 list of important, easy-to-understand facts for patients about stem cell treatments' written by a stem cell scientist on a popular stem cell advisory blog (File4). Only five (of 35) times 'FDA' appeared alongside a positive view. This suggests that the erosion of trust from the perceived conflicts of interest around institutions that legitimise scientific evidence such as the FDA had motivated trust for therapies distrusted by those institutions. As one user noted:

Just because it is 'unproven' by FDA standards does not make it a scam. … Everyone should do their homework and do what is best for themselves. (File2-October/2015)

Thus, if the negative label of 'unproven' frames public trust in eSCTs within the boundaries of scientific evidence and delegitimises those stepping beyond them, then questioning that label (as in the quote above) reflect at the very least (a) cognisance among participants about other ways of knowing or 'proving' and (b) agency to evaluate who can(not) be trusted. Intuitively, that this evidence evaluation was conducted in online communities almost devoid of provider inputs, revealed user-distrust in most providers as self-serving rather than public interest serving:

… 'experts' voiced the concern that so many people trusted you tube more that the CDC FDA etc. That is the problem we don't trust officialdom. … XXX's survey … suggested only one percent of us trust officialdom. (File3-December/2011)

The result of this is a form of user-to-user engagement that is unlike traditional provider–user models of participation premised on providers sharing power with users. Indeed, participants extended and attributed their distrust of providers onto experts by insinuating their collusion with 'Big Pharma' through examples reflecting conflicts of interest; especially targeting experts highly active in calling for global regulatory strengthening against eSCTs. For instance, one participant accused the provider and site-owner of a popular discussion forum of such conflicts of interest:

Doing the work that you do, you are too sophisticated to be ignorant of the actions of the FDA in serving Big Pharma and Big Medicine at the expense of the patient. The only possible explanation for your statements is your collusion and/or your financial dependence. Your statements betray you. (File4-January/2012)

In sum, participants' evaluations of evidence were shaped by distrust in the commitment of EBM's institutions to protecting public interests, especially those individuals and institutions with private or commercial interests. This distrust followed from the reverse logic that if 'unproven' SCTs were demonised by 'untrustworthy' providers, then eSCT practitioners could not be in collusion with Big Pharma – and thus they were worthy of re-evaluation and possibly worthy of trust as well. A key part of this logic was to establish the untrustworthiness of some providers, and this was done by citing instances of provider–industry collusion, corruption among scientific insiders and by discrediting expert credentials with proof of conflicts of interest (File2, File4). This suggests that distrust in some providers motivated some participants to step beyond the provider-constructed definition of eSCTs to evaluate all available evidence for themselves. Notably, distrust in providers is not the only reason that motivates user choice of eSCTs but adds to a host of complex and diverse reasons like illness severity, access restrictions to treatments, etc. explored elsewhere (see, e.g. Salter, Zhou, & Datta, 2014).

How users evaluate evidence

Participants evaluated a range of available evidence, including physicians' advice, experiential evidence and scientific literature. For instance, the discussion threads on *The Niche* and *MS Society UK* mentioned 'published/publication/pub-med' 11 and 14 times respectively (File4 and File3). One participant offered the following sources (at times with hyperlinks) to help other participants to research treatment choices in Multiple Sclerosis (MS):

> … UK-NICE [guidance document]; Centonze etc. of University Hospital Tor Vergata (Rome); the Annals of Neurology, July 2011 (pub-med), MS Matters, Pub-Med (4 times), UK Parliament publications, Cochrane Summary and Monto et.al Report 2008 (IEP.org). (File3-October/2011)

Apart from the scientific research articles discussed above, participants also expressed trust in publications by entities such as the *Cochrane Collaboration*,[4] which provides reviews of diverse conditions based on aggregates of diverse evidence. Overall, participant comments revealed high degrees of trust in basic research papers and publications from sources perceived as trustworthy like *UK Parliament* papers and *Cochrane Collaboration* analyses.

Participants were interested in educating themselves in the science of MS by extensively and exhaustively triangulating their knowledge through searching, monitoring, researching and at times following basic research study results (e.g. cohort studies) over years, often remarking: '… I have researched so much …' or 'I have been researching this for a while and reading on everything I can' (File2-October/2015). One outcome of this was that discussion forums of large disease societies and patient organisations were used by users as knowledge repositories to share and learn about competing views, new research, on-going trial information, members' disease progress (or recovery) and more. In turn, participants used this resource to evaluate media coverage of 'unproven' eSCTs. As one participant commented,

> All too often new treatments are 'glamourised' – there is nothing easy or fool proof! (File2-October/2015)

Some participants also expressed a preference for reading scientific findings informing media coverage (File3-October/2011). Thus suggesting critical evaluation of evidence amongst users that challenge assumptions of information deficit underlying 'gullible' user choices of eSCTs (Master & Resnik, 2011).

Participants requested, shared and empathised with other users' views, evaluations and disease experiences. The *Facebook* page of the *National MS Society* (USA) was one of the most frequently searched pages under the search term MS and contained 15 requests for information about eSCTs. Below is a typical solicitation for further information on discussion forums:

> Hello All, I have recently come across a treatment for MS - CCVSI. It is an operation, which unblocks veins to allow blood flow. It isn't available in the UK but can be done in Poland and some other countries. Has anyone else heard anything or had this treatment???? (File3-October/2011)

The solicitation elicited 67 comments, including five comments about disease experiences and four about 'collusion between pharma and regulators'. It also included 24 comments *for* and 26 *against* experimental therapies. Thus, it was not the case that users only shared or heard 'positive' experiences. On the contrary, users had a high awareness of the risks of eSCTs and evaluated therapies based on individual risk-rationalisation calculus' typically combining low tolerance for 'safety' risks with high preference for 'efficacy' risks as below,

> I have been researching this for a while and reading on everything I can the death rate is less than 1%. (Evaluating 'safety risks'; File2-October/2015)

> … the acceptable risk to the NHS is 1%, the risk so far for the CCSVI intervention is about 100 times lower than that. Some 30,000 people world wide have been treated, only three people have died and a handful have suffered some complications. (Evaluating 'efficacy risks'; File3-October/2011)

Consequently, participants viewed eSCTs as a way of 'improving' quality of life while 'hoping' for cures. The discussion thread on *National MS Society* contained 32 (of 358) posts expressing hope and prayers for a future cure, 23 posts expecting stem cells to improve quality of life and zero comments indicating expectations of a cure from eSCTs. Similarly, while patients expressed trust in eSCTs and wanted others to trust in them, they were careful to convey realistic expectations:

> Like anything else, HSCT doesn't work for 100% of patients, but it works for a very high percentage. (File2-June/2015)

What works for one doesn't for another. No two cases [are] alike as [X] said. … Just don't turn people off from something that may work wonders for them. (File2-October/2015)

Negative views or experiences were shared and viewed as important in participants' evaluations of evidence. As one commented:

… it doesn't work for everyone, and it certainly doesn't do the sort of things that you have a tendency to claim because people DO relapse and DO progress while on it; in fact some people get a lot worse. (File3-December/2011)

Users, in turn, suggested bolstering eSCTs with mainstream medication and wellness regimes for improved results:

Every single person has to find their 'combo'. One size does not fit all … Genetic, vaccine, diet and environment play a part. … It [i.e. HSCT] requires 35 + treatments to be effective. I was treating a frontal lobe brain injury, MS and migraines = gave me a new life! (File2-June/2016)

These conversations highlight the simplistic nature of the view that 'unproven' therapies victimise users who are thought to be gullible (Qiu, 2009) and lacking the capacity to make good health choices without provider intervention (Master & Resnik, 2011). Participants not only conducted exhaustive reviews of disease-specific evidence but made rationalisations of risks and benefits in their individual cases. Indeed, the finding that users access an array of information is consistent with Sharpe et al.'s (2016, p. 445) finding that users engage in 'multi-level information-seeking'. This, in turn, questions the provider presupposition that 'the portrayal of stem cell medicine on provider websites [as] optimistic and unsubstantiated by peer-reviewed literature' may lead users to make poor treatment choices (Lau et al., 2008). For it assumes weak user decision-making processes mostly informed by and dependent on positive provider feedback without considering the complexity and array of sources that users reference.

However, what is conspicuous by its absence (in the conversations analysed here) is the reference to provider-created public advisories warning users against undertaking eSCTs as well as academic papers by bioethicists or sociologists. This absence suggests that users rely on evaluating basic research evidence themselves or its interpretations by large credible bodies with public accountability (e.g. UK Parliament reports) and experiential data from other participants. Indeed, provider constructions of what constitutes 'evidence' (e.g. in provider-run online public advisories warning users against 'unproven' therapies) did not constitute a part of users' evidence base (as shown in the previous section). This suggests that users appeared to have strong trust in basic research findings but not in provider constructed interpretations of its significance for them. At the same time, users placed a high value on experiential data shared in user-to-user settings when evaluating the trustworthiness of evidence for eSCTs. The latter is not surprising because studies show high degrees of trust in small-group 'community' settings when people know each other and where there are fewer chances of 'free-ridership' and 'cheating' (Artinger & Vulkan, 2016; Dietz, Ostrom, & Stern, 2003).

Conclusion

In this paper, I explored why and how people are evaluating 'evidence' themselves through online user-to-user engagement. First, I showed that users' choice to evaluate evidence for themselves is grounded in deep distrust in some provider's commitment to protecting public interests. The underlying logic is that if the untrustworthy institution's distrust 'unproven' therapies then eSCTs are at least worthy of evaluation and possibly worthy of trust as well. This trust for eSCTs also points towards the underlying logic of why user-to-user engagement excludes providers who are viewed as untrustworthy. Second, I showed that distrust in providers could not be conflated with distrust for scientific evidence. On the contrary, users demonstrated high levels of trust in (a) basic research evidence (but not in provider constructed interpretation of its significance for them) and (b) experiential data shared between participants in user-to-user conversations. In effect, this article casts online user-to-user communities as productive epistemic spaces that are challenging the view propagated by providers that scientific evidence is the only legitimate form of knowing or 'proving' therapies. As I have shown, users combine abstract scientific evidence with lived experiences in complex and unpredictable ways. This shifting public perception of what counts as evidence and public trust for who says what counts as evidence not only calls for greater objectivity in presenting clinical evidence as one among many ways of knowing but also for greater user control over upstream evidence generation (Wynne, 2006; Lambert, 2013).

That people trust people and rely on forming an opinion from a wide array of evidence as the data suggest, rather than blindly trust provider constructions of evidence, is evident. In turn, this highlights the shifting relations between the institutions of EBM and society, in which lay people are exerting greater control over the evidence that lies at the heart of evidence-based drug development policies. For if users are increasingly making their own evaluations of evidence with the result that they not only trust eSCTs but are accessing them by travelling beyond the jurisdiction of Euro-American policies that prevent and dissuade access to eSCTs, then for these users at least, these policies have little relevance. This implies that for providers to remain in touch with publics there needs to be greater inclusiveness in the ways in which upstream institutions of EBM engage with users.

Notes

1. Search included substituting 'therapies' with 'treatments'.
2. http://css.csail.mit.edu/6.858/2014/readings/sybilrank.pdf.
3. US-based private clinic offering eSCTs for orthopaedic conditions.
4. http://www.cochrane.org/CD009956/MS_exercise-therapy-fatigue-multiple-sclerosis

Acknowlegement

I would like to thank Salla Sariola: University of Turku and University of Oxford, Lindsey Reynolds Stellenbosch University and Brown University, and Justin Dixon: University of Durham for their helpful suggestions and insight in shaping this research paper.

Disclosure statement

The author reports no conflict of interest.

Funding

This work was supported by the UK's Economic and Social Research Council [grant number ES/J012521/1].

ORCID

Saheli Datta ⓘ http://orcid.org/0000-0001-8268-9013

References

Andreassen, H., & Trondsen, M. (2010). The empowered patient and the sociologist. *Social Theory & Health, 8*(3), 280–287.

Artinger, S., & Vulkan, N. (2016). Does group size matter for behavior in online trust dilemmas? *PLoS ONE, 11*(11), e0166279.

Aubusson, K. (2014). GP used stem cell therapy in autism. *Australian Doctor*. Retrieved from https://www.australiandoctor.com.au/news/gp-used-stem-cell-therapy-autism

Bazzano, A. N., Martin, J., Hicks, E., Faughnan, M., & Murphy, L. (2017). Human-centred design in global health: A scoping review of applications and contexts. *PLoS ONE, 12*(11), e0186744.

Beninger, K., Fry, A., Jago, N., Lepps, H., Nass, L., & Silvester, H. (2014). Social media; users' views. *NatCen Social Research, 1*–40.

Berger, I., Ahmad, A., Bansal, A., Kapoor, T., Sipp, D., & Rasko, J. E. J. (2016). Global distribution of businesses marketing stem cell-based interventions. *Cell Stem Cell, 19*(2), 158–162.

Bharadwaj, A. (2012). Enculturating cells: The anthropology, substance, and science of stem cells. *Annual Review of Anthropology, 41*, 303–317.

Brennan, Z. (2017). Senate passes 'right-to-try' bill. *Regulatory Affairs Professional Society*. Retrieved from http://www.raps.org/Regulatory-Focus/News/2017/08/03/28171/ Senate-Passes-Right-to-Try-Bill/

Cao, Q., Sirivianos, M., Yang, X., & Pregueiro, T. (2012). Aiding the detection of fake accounts in large scale social online services. In *Proceedings of the 9th USENIX Conference on Networked Systems Design and Implementation* (pp. 1–14). Berkeley, CA: USENIX Association.

Charles, C., Gafni, A., & Freeman, E. (2011). The evidence-based medicine model of clinical practice: Scientific teaching or belief-based preaching? *Journal of Evaluation in Clinical Practice, 17*(4), 597–605.

Chen, H., & Gottweis, H. (2013). Stem cell treatments in China: Rethinking the patient role in the global bio-economy. *Bioethics, 27*(4), 194–207.

Dietz, T., Ostrom, E., & Stern, P. C. (2003). The struggle to govern the commons. *Science, 302*(5652), 1907–1912.

Djulbegovic, B., Guyatt, G. H., & Ashcroft, R. E. (2009). Epistemologic inquiries in evidence-based medicine. *Cancer Control, 16*(2), 158–168.

Dresser, R. (2014). The right to try investigational drugs: Science and stories in the access debate. *Texas Law Review, 93*, 1631–1657.

Eisenstein, M. (2016). Regulation: Rewriting the regenerative rulebook. *Nature, 540*(7632), S64–S67.

Epstein, S. (1996). *Impure science: AIDS, activism, and the politics of knowledge* (Vol. 7). Berkeley: University of California Press.

Facey, K., Boivin, A., Gracia, J., Hansen, H. P., Scalzo, A. L., Mossman, J., & Single, A. (2010). Patients' perspectives in health technology assessment: A route to robust evidence and fair deliberation. *International Journal of Technology Assessment in Health Care, 26*(3), 334–340.

Foster, D. (2016). 'Keep complaining til someone listens': Exchanges of tacit healthcare knowledge in online illness communities. *Social Science & Medicine, 166*, 25–32.

Greenhalgh, T., Snow, R., Ryan, S., Rees, S., & Salisbury, H. (2015). Six 'biases' against patients and carers in evidence-based medicine. *BMC Medicine, 13*(1), 86–210.

Haas, P. M. (2001). Policy knowledge: Epistemic communities. In N. J. Smelser & B. Baltes (Eds.), *International encyclopedia of the social & behavioral sciences* (pp. 11578–11586). Oxford: Elsevier.

Hyysalo, S., & Johnson, M. (2015). The user as relational entity. *Information Technology & People, 28*(1), 72–89.

ISSCR. (2008). Guidelines for the clinical translation of stem cells. *International Sociey for Stem Cell Research*. Retrieved from http://www.isscr.org/docs/default-source/all-isscr-guidelines/clin-trans-guidelines/isscrglclinicaltrans.pdf?sfvrsn=6

ISSCR. (2013). ISSCR voices concern as Italian government authorizes unproven stem cell therapy. *International Sociey for Stem Cell Research*. Retrieved from http://www.isscr.org/home/about-us/news-press-releases/2013/2013/04/10/isscr-voices-concern-as-italian-government-authorizes-unproven-stem-cell-therapy

Kallinikos, J., & Tempini, N. (2014). Patient data as medical facts: Social media practices as a foundation for medical knowledge creation. *Information Systems Research, 25*(4), 817–833.

Lambert, H. (2013). Plural forms of evidence in public health: Tolerating epistemological and methodological diversity. *Evidence & Policy, 9*(1), 43–48.

Lau, D., Ogbogu, U., Taylor, B., Stafinski, T., Menon, D., & Caulfield, T. (2008). Stem cell clinics online: The direct-to-consumer portrayal of stem cell medicine. *Cell Stem Cell, 3*(6), 591–594.

Leach, M., Scoones, I., & Wynne, B. (2005). *Science and citizens: Globalization and the challenge of engagement* (Vol. 2). London: Zed Books.

Lupton, D. (2013). The digitally engaged patient: Self-monitoring and self-care in the digital health era. *Social Theory & Health, 11*(3), 256–270.

Markham, A., & Buchannan, E. (2012). Ethical decision- making and internet research: Recommendations from the AoIR Ethics Working Committee. *Association of Internet Researchers (AoIR)*. Retrieved from http://aoir.org/reports/ethics2.pdf

Master, Z., & Resnik, D.B. (2011). Stem-cell tourism and scientific responsibility. *EMBO Reports, 12*(10), 992–995.

Matthews, K. R. W., & Iltis, A. S. (2015). Unproven stem cell-based interventions and achieving a compromise policy among the multiple stakeholders. *BMC Medical Ethics, 16*(1), 75–85.

McLean, A. K., Stewart, C., & Kerridge, I. (2015). Untested, unproven, and unethical: The promotion and provision of autologous stem cell therapies in Australia. *Stem Cell Research & Therapy, 6*(1), 12–20.

Miles, A., & Mezzich, J. (2011). The care of the patient and the soul of the clinic: Person-centered medicine as an emergent model of modern clinical practice. *The International Journal of Person Centered Medicine, 1*(2), 207–222.

Pear, R., & Kaplan, S. (2017). Senate passes F.D.A. funding and 'right to try' drug bills. *The New York Times*. Retrieved from https://www.nytimes.com/2017/08/03/us/politics/fda-senate-experimental-drugs-terminally-ill-patients.html?mcubz=1

Petersen, A., MacGregor, C., & Munsie, M. (2016). Stem cell miracles or Russian roulette?: Patients' use of digital media to campaign for access to clinically unproven treatments. *Health, Risk and Society, 17*(7–8), 592–604.

Pew Research-Fox, S., & Duggan, M. (2013). Health online 2013. *Pew Research*. Retrieved from http://www.pewinternet.org/2013/01/15/health-online-2013/

PricewaterhouseCoopers. (2012). Social media 'likes' healthcare. *PWC Health Research Institute*. Retrieved from https://www.pwc.com/us/en/health-industries/health-research-institute/publications/pdf/health-care-social-media-report.pdf

Putnam, R. D. (1993). The prosperous community. *The American Prospect, 4*(13), 35–42.

Qiu, J. (2009). Trading on hope. *Nature Biotechnology, 27*(9), 790–792.

Rachul, C. (2011). 'What have I got to lose?': An analysis of stem cell therapy patients' blogs. *Health Law Review, 20*(1), 5–12.

Ramesh, R. (2005). Row over doctor's 'miracle cures'. *The Guardian*. Retrieved from https://www.theguardian.com/science/2005/nov/18/stemcells.controversiesinscience

Salter, B., Zhou, Y., & Datta, S. (2014). Making choices: Health consumers, regulation and the global stem cell therapy market. *Biodrugs, 28*(5), 461–464.

Salter, B., Zhou, Y., & Datta, S. (2015). Hegemony in the marketplace of biomedical innovation: Consumer demand and stem cell science. *Social Science & Medicine, 131*, 156–163.

Sharpe, K., Di Pietro, N., Jacob, K. J., & Illes, J. (2016). A dichotomy of information-seeking and information-trusting: Stem cell interventions and children with neurodevelopmental disorders. *Stem Cell Reviews and Reports, 12*(4), 438–447.

Smith, R.C., Bossen, C., & Kanstrup, A. M. (2017). Participatory design in an era of participation. *CoDesign, 13*(2), 65–69.

Starr, P. (1982). The social origins of professional sovereignty. In *The social transformation of american medicine* (pp. 13–29). New York, NY: Basic Books Inc.

Tonelli, M. R. (2006). Integrating evidence into clinical practice: An alternative to evidence-based approaches. *Journal of Evaluation in Clinical Practice, 12*(3), 248–256.

Turner, L., & Knoepfler, P. (2016). Selling stem cells in the USA: Assessing the direct-to-consumer industry. *Cell Stem Cell, 19*(2), 154–157.

Wright, S., & Street, J. (2007). Democracy, deliberation and design: The case of online discussion forums. *New Media & Society, 9*(5), 849–869.

Wynne, B. (2006). Public engagement as a means of restoring public trust in science – Hitting the notes, but missing the music? *Community Genetics, 9*(3), 211–220.

The possibility of addressing epistemic injustice through engaged research practice: reflections on a menstruation related critical health education project in South Africa

Sharli Anne Paphitis

ABSTRACT

Questions of epistemic injustice in relation to community engagement activities have rarely been interrogated. While it is often purported that when academics and community members are involved in the co-creation of knowledge through a mutually beneficial exchange of resources and expertise, all participants emerge as active stakeholders in the knowledge production process, little research has been done on how academics or community partners experience these processes from an epistemological perspective. Does the proposed process of repositioning research participants in community engagement praxis allows for a new power dynamic to emerge in research such that all parties genuinely share equal responsibility for determining the processes and outcomes of the knowledge production process? Do such activities allow for an epistemological shift away from traditional knowledge construction paradigms to ones in which the democratisation of knowledge is prioritised? Does such an epistemological shift in the knowledge construction paradigm extend beyond simply the knowledge construction process to interpersonal relationships between academics and community members who see themselves as co-protagonists in a shared project? In grappling with these questions I will draw on my own, personal experiences working in a menstruation related engaged research critical health education project in South Africa, to discuss the complexities of whether and how the amelioration of epistemic injustices are being served through community engagement activities.

Epistemic injustice and engaged research

Given the post-apartheid calls for the transformation of the South African higher education sector at the level of policy directives, as well as the real and pressing need for issues of social justice, decolonisation and redress that face all sectors of South African society, it is surprising to find that higher education transformation 'has not shown as much progress as might be expected' (Erasmus, 2014, p. 105). Recent student-led movements (in particular the #RhodesMustFall and #FeesMustFall protests) have called for the decolonisation of South African higher education institutions and the democratisation of the knowledge production process. Student movements have raised important questions about the accessibility and relevance of academic knowledge, as well as questions of epistemic justice with regards to whose knowledge counts within the academy. Much of the literature stemming from the debates in social epistemology focus on defining the concept of epistemic *injustice* much more explicitly than epistemic *justice*. Within this piece, I take epistemic justice to refer to both the principles governing epistemic systems and engagements (as per Anderson, 2012), as well as the normative idea, as suggested by Glass and Newman (2015), that epistemic activity ought to follow principles of fairness, cooperation and mutual respect. The above-mentioned questions raised in student movements intersect with the challenges raised by community engagement theorists (Glass & Newman, 2015; Leblanc & Kinsella, 2016), who have recently grappled with questions of epistemic (in)justice within the higher education sector, and in particular, epistemic practices with respect to research conducted with the communities in which they are situated. Within this community engagement literature, it has been suggested that adopting particular research practices allows institutions and those who work there to perpetuate epistemic injustices as they 'subtly – and not so subtly – *ignore and discredit* ways of knowing and understanding the world' (Bernal & Villalpando, 2002, p. 169) that those from non-privileged groups bring.

An epistemic injustice can be understood a kind of harm in which individuals or groups are wronged in their capacity as bearers of knowledge, or as 'knowers', or as epistemic agents (Fricker, 2007). Epistemic injustices are those which dehumanise groups as well as individuals by delegitimising them as knowers – either in the eyes of society or the academy, or their own eyes. Epistemic injustice is committed both when agents are barred from having their testimony enter the marketplace of ideas, and when an 'active epistemic agent (or subject)' is relegated 'to that of passive object, to be studied, observed, and in many cases, exploited' (LeBlanc & Kinsella, 2016, p. 66). Further, epistemic injustice accrues when marginalised or oppressed individuals or groups struggle to interpret the world and their place in it, without having to do so through lenses constructed by dominant or powerful groups whose perspectives, meanings and discourse are at best 'ill-fitting' and, at worst, render those individual's or group's experiences quite unintelligible from an insiders perspective (Fricker, 2007, p. 149). Here, Glass and Newman (2015) suggest that the individuals and groups whose knowledge is systematically undermined through epistemic prejudice are not only barred from reinterpreting the world for themselves, but more importantly, they stress that they are barred from being given the opportunity to do so for others.

Since academic and research epistemic communities enjoy privileged epistemic positions in society, they already and necessarily operate from a position of power and privilege when they engage with broader society. Particularly in research settings, participants are seen as lacking the epistemic credibility of their 'epistemically privileged counterparts', namely the researchers (Leblanc & Kinsella, 2016; Medina, 2012). Most problematically, in the higher education sector such biases serve to further marginalise the voices and testimony of individuals and groups whose 'knowledge claims enter the marketplace of ideas at a very substantial disadvantage,' (Glass & Newman, 2015, p. 27) when they are being received by, evaluated and assessed by, and assimilated into frameworks and paradigms determined by (for the most part) hearers from dominant groups.

The mandate for community engagement in South Africa, particularly through engaged research endeavours, has been to transform the sector by breaking down the division between town and gown and to make academe more socially responsive and accessible. The ultimate aim has been to democratise the knowledge economy – which is still largely divided along socio-economic and racial lines owing to the legacy of apartheid. Community engagement, particularly in the form of engaged research (encompassing a broad range of methodological approaches, arguably on a spectrum of engagement,[1] such as community-based participatory research, community-based research, and participatory action research) ostensibly allows for the co-creation of knowledge between communities and researchers involved in mutually beneficial research partnerships. Proponents of engaged research argue that this methodological approach provides an important avenue for academics and institutions to conduct their research in more socially responsive, democratic and participatory ways (Blumenthal, 2011; Cook, 2008; Israel, Schulz, Parker, & Becker, 1998; Michener et al., 2012; Sofolahan-Oladeinde, Mullins, & Baquet, 2015).

The term 'participation' within this context warrants exploration and discussion. Within the literature and debates in development studies in particular, the term participation has become contentious, and seen as a 'buzz word', given the misappropriation of the term for political or ideological agendas.

Participation has, in many projects been used as synonymous with mere consultation. Within this context, it is important to ask what participation within a research project could, or perhaps should, amount to? Arguably, as with engagement, participation could occur within a spectrum depending on the project, the goals and the methodology employed. At a minimum, participation requires the active involvement of participants in the research project, where being active would amount to participants understanding the research project, as well as commitment to and investment in at least some of the research process and outcomes. But, I think the underlying principles driving what can be seen as 'participatory research' requires researchers to problematise the power differentials of research by fully involve their participants in the research processes which are, often unreflectively, conducted 'independently' and which are typically inaccessible to participants. The challenges arising from this new way of doing research are a source for rich debate. Participatory research as central to engaged research processes, and aligning with the goals of addressing epistemic justice through engagement, strive to bring out the strengths of researchers and 'participants' as they work in a partnership for research through which the balance of power inherent in the knowledge generation process is challenged (see Horowitz, Robinson, & Seifer, 2009 for a discussion of participation in these terms).

Following this, engaged research, at least in principle, provides an important way for higher education institutions to challenge and undermine epistemic injustices by respecting individuals and communities outside of the traditional academic boundaries as 'knowledge-bearers', 'knowledge producers' and participants in the research process in a very real sense, rather than merely 'research subjects' sources of data or knowledge recipients (Glass & Newman, 2015, p. 32). Perhaps most importantly, engaged research is built on the normative principle of what Visvanathan has called cognitive justice[2]: embracing a plurality of knowledges from diverse perspectives of legitimate epistemic agents who enter into dialogue with one another within a research relationship (Davies, 2016). Through the promotion of cognitive/epistemic justice, engaged research practices opening up the knowledge economy to those who were previously barred from playing an active role in it.

Globally engaged research is still subject to significant scepticism by those who continue to raise debates about the 'bias of various sorts of justificatory warrants, and about the specific forms of knowledge and understanding authorized by universities' (Glass & Newman, 2015, p. 33, see also Karnilowicz, Ali, & Phillimore, 2014). Debate and critical inquiry on the topic of engagement is important if the goals of epistemic justice are to be advanced, and it is important for academics to recognise their own biases and prejudices in the project of re-imagining their own and other's roles in the knowledge production process. In South Africa, community engagement (understood as mutually beneficial activities done in partnership with local communities[3]) has yet to become institutionalised, despite the important role these activities would have in increasing the social responsiveness of the sector. Given that epistemic value is undoubtedly found not only within academic or dominant communities, it is concerning that South African scholars on engagement have cautioned that 'some local academics have come to the conclusion that what lies beyond the ivory tower is an "intellectual wasteland"' (Erasmus, 2014, p. 107).

Potts and Brown (2005) have argued that the process of engaged research 'can be emancipating, community building, a catalyst for social change, and a starting point for some serious self-discovery' (p. 257). They have also pointed out that as we work for societal change through engaged research 'we recognize that usually the first target of change is ourselves' (p. 260). In writing this paper, I aim to reflect on my own experiences working in an engaged research project in an effort to unpack and explore my own developments as an academic and researcher, as well as my own evolving processes of epistemic transformation as they unfolded. In reflecting on my experiences, I also aim to explore the epistemic shifts and transformations – as well as what I perceived as barriers to these – in my colleagues and community partners as we worked through the various stages of this project. I hope that my reflections may serve as a catalyst to prompt further debate, shared reflective practice of this kind from researchers through which we might draw deeper collective wisdom.

Siyahluma: *we* need to conduct a needs assessment

My reflections which follow stem from my work over three years in a critical health education research and intervention project – *Siyahluma* ('We are growing') – and aim to stimulate further thought and debate about the nature of engagement, participation and epistemic justice in a knowledge generation process. The project centred on addressing the challenges faced by school-going girls in relation to menstruation (see similar issues reported in Grant, Lloyd, & Mensch, 2013; Kirk & Sommer, 2006; Mason et al., 2013; Tegegne & Sisay, 2014; Vaughn, 2013). In the first instance, the project sought to establish what the sources of knowledge about menstruation for school-going girls across the Eastern Cape (South Africa) were, what practices were being used for menstrual management in schools, and whether menstruation negatively affected school attendance. The project also aimed to address not only the lack of access to reliable and affordable sanitary products (through the distribution of reusable and disposable sanitary products made by a local woman's sewing group working in partnership with our research team), but also a lack of access to non-stigmatised[4] information about menstruation in local schools through education intervention projects run in partnership with local NGO's and schools.

The concern that school-going girls were not able to afford sanitary products, and were thus unable to attend school while menstruating, was raised and brought to my attention by one of my University's community partner organisations. After the initial expression of concern from the community partner, however, a meeting was held between various academic stakeholders where it was decided that 'we need to conduct a needs assessment survey'. We, the academics, set out to design questionnaires which would be distributed at a cross-section of high schools across our province to address important questions such as: 'what is the relationship between access to menstrual products and absenteeism from school?'; 'what is the relationship between access to knowledge about menstruation and absenteeism from school?'; and 'what stigmas and taboos are associated with menstruation?'. At the end of this process we had drafted a 16 page survey aimed at penultimate high school level female learners, received institutional ethics approval and distributed the survey to 20 schools across the province (a process which took well over a year).

In critically reflecting on the methods we had employed to conduct the needs assessment, what became apparent to me was that the framing of our overall questions positioned us outside, rather than inside of the research – by asking for example 'what stigmas and taboos are associated with menstruation?', as opposed to 'how can we work together to address the stigmas and taboos associated with menstruation?'. As I began to reflect, I started to recognise that although the project was perceived both from within and without to be an engaged research project (based on the fact that the initial need had identified by the local community, the research topic was responding to an issue of local concern,[5] and there was a plan – however vague at that stage – for some action or change to be implemented through the research), there was little about the project that could be said to be, at that time, genuinely participatory. For the most part we were seeking to establish theories and frameworks for our research subjects about their situation, without treating them as epistemic agents in their own right, capable of playing a role in the knowledge economy. As such, the project could hardly be said to be changing the relationship between the subjects of the research and ourselves, let alone undermining the assumption that we, the researchers, were ultimately the producers of knowledge within the project (Pizarro, 1998; Potts & Brown, 2005). Our needs assessment survey was primarily aimed at uncovering things as they 'really' are – in an effort to provide an objective and scientific report, from our academic analysis and perspective, on the extent of the problems around menstruation in the local community, rather than bringing out and showcasing the different voices, knowledges and perspectives already available from those in our local community around the topic of menstruation. We had neither engaged with our community (in particular, school learners) in constructing our survey, nor involved them in the data collection or analysis process, and while we had meaningful interactions with educators at the schools, this had not formed part of the formal research process. The locus of power thus remained firmly in our, rather than the participant's, hands.

In light of all this, I began to unpack, more critically, that significant 'but' utterance, 'but *we* need to conduct a needs assessment'. While we had not ignored the insight brought to us by the catalysing community partner altogether, there is certainly something disturbing about the fact that the 'we' in this statement implicitly referred only to us as university researchers. It somehow excluded that community partner from the knowledge generation process and that certainly seems to delegitimise their knowledge claim, as well as undervalue them as epistemic agents and their role in the knowledge production process. Certainly, I am not suggesting that the mere report by this community partner should have been taken as absolute knowledge, and I am not thus dismissing the importance of a needs assessment. Insider perspectives and reports of situations should be seen as catalysts for further exploration into reported knowledges, findings, perspectives, and situations in ways which ideally allow for the dialogical analysis of that knowledge. Reflecting on this preliminary stage of the project, however, certainly forced me to ask some important, more general questions about epistemic justice in the knowledge generation process.

Particularly in the construction of our surveys, it seems that we as researchers had largely ignored the epistemic agency of the participants who were providing us with what we were largely seeing as data, rather than knowledge, and we saw our own role in analysing this 'raw' data as the knowledge generation process. In our work with partner schools there was little resistance to our approach. No questions were raised about how were going about the work that we were doing, how we would report back on our findings or if there were more collaborative ways in which we could be working to either generate the knowledge or implement programmes which would result. At this stage of the research, we had little understanding of our position of relative privilege in respect to the knowledge creation process. We did not recognise that our own approaches to our interactions with community members and partners could shape their relative ability to see themselves as internal to the research and thus being able to challenge, critique or add to the research process itself. In using what we saw as data from our participants, we aimed to construct knowledge that we would use to build programmes that we saw as the 'participatory part' of the project which would speak to their situations and experiences through our analyses – but which we had ultimately constructed from our own interpretive paradigm. Rather than constructing an action intervention project in which we allowed our target group to make their own critiques and ideas visible, we were working in isolation from those who we, for the most part implicitly, assumed lacked the interpretative resources to both critique the situation and, working collaboratively, formulate intervention plans to address them. In doing this we were, I suggest, implicitly, though unintentionally, perpetuating epistemic injustices.

In light of this, we began to re-evaluate how the research project should continue. In thinking through how we wanted to move forward in the project, we came to see that we needed to immerse ourselves more fully in partnerships with community based organisations and local schools to create mutual goals and a knowledge sharing network – removing ourselves even further from the role of 'disinterested' researchers and at times even come to blur the lines between researchers and activists within the project (Temper & Bene, 2016). In doing this we hoped to achieve a project in which members of traditionally marginalised or oppressed groups[6] would be given opportunities, resources and platforms to interpret their experiences of the world for themselves and others and to share these interpretations with hearers who give such interpretations credence.

Sharing knowledge, constructing knowledge and participatory community health education interventions

In what follows, I briefly reflect on the two health education intervention projects we undertook after adopting a more collaborative approach to the project, highlighting the ways in which our methodological and epistemological practices and views evolved from the initial stages of this research project. These reflections aim to highlight some of the ways in which more participatory approaches could arguably allow for the democratisation of the knowledge production process, as well as allowing for traditionally marginalised voices of to emerge more strongly in the knowledge construction and dissemination process.

In immersing ourselves in the engaged research process, we decided to bring together a number of local NGOs and schools to work as part of a collective in designing critical health education interventions on menstruation. Bringing together a number of diverse stakeholders in what turned out to be a forum-like space allowed us to share our inputs and perspectives, while listening to the views and opinions of a diverse array of people. We found ourselves deferring to their expertise on many occasions in issues related to how to go about running various interventions, and through this process came to challenge many of our own 'unexamined assumptions of authority and expertise' (Sohng, 1996, p. 87). As a collective we agreed to implement two major health education interventions which were distinct, though interrelated – the first in the form of interactive workshop sessions in schools and the second in the form of a community theatre project. Our work in these health education interventions marked a major turning point in our approach to the research project. The project was no longer about collecting data to generate knowledge. Rather, we saw ourselves as involved in an emerging and political process of co-creating knowledge with our participants. We saw our interventions themselves as part of the knowledge-making cycle. In this cycle, we, along with our partners and our participants, would be able to grapple with, learn more about, and come to make sense of the issues we were ultimately trying to address through our interventions *collectively*.

The first health education intervention was done in collaboration with a local NGO employing social workers who run life orientation classes in schools, and involved us collaboratively workshopping and re-curriculating a section of their life-skills programme which dealt with issues of puberty and sexuality. While we brought much of our research to bear on the re-curriculation process, we relied on the expertise and skills of the social workers in transforming this into a series of interactive workshops rather than lessons. As we worked through this process of re-curriculation, our interdependence on each other's equally vital skills and expertise showed a marked shift in our research method to one which was becoming increasingly dialogical. This dialogical relationship between the social workers and ourselves began to take on a more democratic dimension as they began to see our work together increasingly as a 'conversation among equals' (van der Reit, 2008, p. 552). By making use of interactive workshops, participants would be involved in not only contributing their own experiences and knowledge to the sessions, but shaping the direction and outcomes of the workshops through dialogue with the facilitators. In this way, participants were able to contribute the structure of the knowledge construction process which was occurring during these workshops, determining which issues within the broader theme were of particular relevance to their experiences and situations, and which they felt most strongly about addressing. While the social workers played a leadership role in facilitating the workshops, a member of our research group assisted them in their facilitation – this marked a shift in the relations of power between ourselves, our partners and our participants, and consequently a shift in our understanding of who was 'controlling' the knowledge generation process at this point in the project.

Similarly, in the second health intervention project we worked in collaboration with a local high school to workshop a community theatre production around menstruation, working with both the drama teacher and school learners. In workshopping the play, learners took control of the knowledge generation process and bore equal responsibility for the outcomes of that process – as essentially the 'owners' of one of most significant knowledge products in the form of an educational play. Since we came to see the play itself as a product of the knowledge production process, it was also seen as one of the iterative results of the knowledge generation process itself. Importantly, in all this our participants had been involved not merely as research subjects or passive recipients at any stage of this process. The play was an important product of the knowledge generation process in which the participants themselves were able to voice their own understandings, meanings and analyses in not only a very public, but also a deeply meaningful way.

Following their performance, the actors hosted a post-performance dialogue session with their audience, which was co-facilitated by teachers and ourselves. In these post-performance dialogues we initially played a more active role in the facilitation, sharing willingly own insights and personal experiences, but as the high school learners gained increased confidence of their own knowledge and expertise, they no longer felt they had to defer to or rely on us in these sessions. This marked a shift in their own understanding of who the 'experts' in the project were, as well as our own, and we came to see that we were moving the knowledge generation and intervention process forward and into the hands of our participants through the active transfer of our skills. As the high school learners became more confident they engaged in deep cooperative meaning making with the shared dialogical space which emerged between the two groups who were engaging in collective process of finding solutions to the challenges expressed through the questions raised in the forum.

Importantly, in both of these critical health education interventions our participants were now made up of both male and female learners, as opposed to the female only population who had filled in the surveys. What this meant was that we were now including more diverse perspectives into the knowledge generation process, and garnering the opinions and experiences of those who we had previously assumed would have had little to contribute to the research question (and this had much to do with the initial framing of that question). In relation to this development of the project in particular it is important to point out that more reflection could also be given here to the general history of epistemic injustice with respect to the production of knowledge about women's bodies.[7] What is noteworthy here is that the shift in our work to more effective forms of participation led to our work operating outside of a narrow gender lens which would relegate menstruation to either a female or biological purview. Given the shift in the project towards a relational approach to gender and the erasure of gender divisions, there is room here, however, for debate and discussion about the kind of participatory approach encouraged in this project in this respect.[8] Since we were now working to establish how we could address the challenges related to menstruation across an intersection of social, economic and cultural realities, it was clear that everyone had a role to play in bringing their understandings, experiences and opinions to bear on how to build solutions collectively within the participant groups, as well as within our community and society more broadly. In short, we began to recognise and respect the epistemic agency of our community partners more fully.

From the analysis presented in my reflections here it may seem clear that my, and my collaborator's, work has led us to understand the relationship between researchers and participants in such a way that epistemic injustice accrues when participants are not actively involved at all stages of the research process (from design, through data generation, analysis and interpretation as well as dissemination). One thing to be debated here would be whether the epistemic injustices perpetrated at each stage in the research process were comparable, and whether or not we might think of research projects as ranging on a scale of participation in which greater epistemic justice was brought about through the knowledge generation process (by having more stages of the research being participatory).

Concluding remarks

In the evolution of our engaged research project we had come a long way in developing participatory practices and approaches, interrogating how we viewed and harnessed the epistemic agency of our participants in the knowledge generation process to further our collective goals for social change. While we had come to recognise the community workshops, theatre initiative and dialogue sessions as important parts of the knowledge generation and knowledge dissemination processes, I think it is still a matter of contention and debate amongst our colleagues in the academy as to whether the legitimacy of these approaches is to be recognised and valued 'academically'. While the aims and the impact of this project was applauded, and indeed celebrated, the initial phase of the research project remained, in most of our colleagues' eyes, the most interesting, valid and valuable aspect of the project in terms of research findings. Similarly, in reporting on the project, the academic outputs (conference papers, reports, book chapters) remained what the institution and funders deemed relevant to the knowledge outputs of the project. We had of course produced these standard and 'legitimate' outputs, though we had not produced any of them collaboratively with our partners or participants. In one instance we had tried to involve our partners in a presentation at the university, but they backed out of participation on the day we were going to present, and although they gave us a number of reasons for this, I still wonder about the explicit or implicit reasons not expressed – whether they saw any value in this activity when they had been so involved in the other community based knowledge dissemination projects which were more participatory in style and directly linked to the local community, or whether they felt intimidated by the academic audience.

Through our engagement with other members of the university community in relation to this project, I have come to doubt that we could fully undermine the scepticism about engaged research and epistemic prejudice through presenting arguments, giving more workshops on what engaged research methodologies entail or even by highlighting and rewarding the positive effects of engaged research projects. I think that much of the work that needs to be done in the academy is to understand how research practices can be harnesses to undo the epistemic injustice that has been perpetuated (and continues to be perpetuated) by academe. From my own experience, achieving this will arguably require a more human face – sharing personal narratives of change through engagement as well as having academics experience these changes themselves through doing, possibly by unwittingly blundering into, community engaged and participatory projects through which they may come to challenge their own ways of being, perceiving and knowing. Perhaps, it will require that we build a critical mass of academics and researchers who not only profess to follow engaged research methodologies, but who take the democratisation of the knowledge production process seriously and who are willing to uncover and reject epistemic injustices in the modern academy. Such academics and researchers are, I think, those who are bold enough to challenge their preconceived ideas, brave enough to constantly interrogate as well as analyse their own practices and refine them in light of critical reflection, and honest enough to learn how to do things differently as they admit to and then confront their mistakes and failures. In seeking to transform how we do our own research, we should, I think, strive to cultivate the kind of 'slow and "care-full" scholarship' (Temper & Bene, 2016, p. 46) as well as academic humility that will allow us to become these kinds of academics. In doing this I suspect that we will also become the kind of academics that community based organisations will be more willing to engage with in meaningful collaborations.

Ethics

Ethical clearance for the project described in this paper was obtained from the Rhodes University Ethical Standards Committee.

Notes

1. The engaged project described in this reflection may indeed have moved from one end of this spectrum to the other as it evolved.
2. Cognitive justice and epistemic justice may be understood as distinct from one another, though should be seen as operating on a spectrum of epistemic harms and goods in relation to recognising the epistemic agency of human beings.
3. Including elements of mutual planning, execution and evaluation of the projects.
4. Much of the information available to school-going girls about menstruation, as identified both in the literature and in our survey, is highly stigmatised: situating menstruation as shameful, surrounded by various myths and taboos.
5. Initially raised by a community based organisation who approached us, but later through the various school principals and teachers we met with while conducting our survey.
6. Particularly in this project, women and children, but more generally community partners in the research process.
7. For some reflections on the ways in which women's knowledge systems are minimised in critical public health projects and literature see Hawkes and Buse (2013) and Burgess (2016).
8. Ethical issues arise in relation to participatory work which brings cultural tension to the fore. For a detailed discussion see Paphitis and Kelland (2018).

Disclosure statement

No potential conflict of interest was reported by the author.

References

Anderson, E. (2012). Epistemic justice as a virtue of social institutions. *Social Epistemology, 26*(2), 163–173.

Bernal, D., & Villalpando, O. (2002). An apartheid of knowledge in academia: The struggle over the "legitimate" knowledge of faculty of color. *Equity and Excellence in Education, 35*(2), 169–180.

Blumenthal, C. (2011). Is community-based participatory research possible? *American Journal of Preventive Medicine, 40*(3), 386–389.

Burgess, R. A. (2016). Dangerous discourses? Silencing women within global mental health practice. In J. Gideon (Ed.), *Handbook on gender and health* (pp. 79–97). Cheltenham: Edward-Elgar Press.

Cook, W. (2008). Integrating research and action: A systematic review of community-based participatory research to address health disparities in environmental and occupational health in the USA. *Journal of Epidemiology & Community Health, 62*(8), 668–676.

Davies, C. (2016). Whose knowledge counts? Exploring cognitive justice in community-university collaborations (PhD Thesis). University of Brighton.

Erasmus, M. (2014). The political unconscious of higher education community engagement in South Africa. In M. Erasmus & R. Albertyn (Eds.), *Knowledge as enablement: Engagement between higher education and the third sector in South Africa* (pp. 100–118). Bloemfontein: Sun Press.

Fricker, M. (2007). *Epistemic injustice: Power and the ethics of knowing.* London: Oxford University Press.

Glass, R., & Newman, A. (2015). Ethical and epistemic dilemmas in knowledge production: Addressing intersection in collaborative, community-based research. *Theory and Research in Education, 13*(1), 23–37.

Grant, M., Lloyd, C., & Mensch, B. (2013). Menstruation and school absenteeism: Evidence from rural Malawi. *Comparative Education Review, 18*(9), 230–284.

Hawkes, S., & Buse, K. (2013). Gender and global health: Evidence, policy, and inconvenient truths. *The Lancet, 381*(9879), 1783–1787.

Horowitz, C., Robinson, M., & Seifer, S. (2009). Community-based participatory research from the margin to the mainstream: are researchers prepared? *Circulation, 119*(19), 2633–2642.

Israel, B. A., Schulz, A. J., Parker, E. A., & Becker, A. B. (1998). Review of community-based research: Assessing partnership approaches to improved public health. *Annual Review of Public Health, 19*, 173–202.

Karnilowicz, W., Ali, L., & Phillimore, J. (2014). Community research within a social constructionist epistemology: Implications for "scientific rigor". *Community Development, 45*(4), 353–367.

Kirk, J., & Sommer, M. (2006). Menstruation and body awareness: Linking girls' health with girls' education. *Tropical Institute (KIT), Special on Gender and Health*, 1–22. Retrieved from http://www.wsscc.org/sites/default/files/publications/kirk-2006-menstruation-kit_paper.pdf\nhttp://www.susana.org/_resources/documents/default/2-1200-kirk-2006-menstruation-kit-paper.pdf

LeBlanc, S., & Kinsella, E. (2016). Toward epistemic justice: A critically reflexive examination of 'sanism' and implications for knowledge generation. *Studies in Social Justice, 10*(1), 59–78.

Mason, L., Nyothach, E., Alexander, K., Odhiambo, F. O., Eleveld, A., Vulule, J., ... Phillips-Howard, P. A. (2013). "We keep it secret so no one should know" – A qualitative study to explore young schoolgirls attitudes and experiences with menstruation in rural Western Kenya. *PLoS One, 8*(11), e79132. doi:10.1371/journal.pone.0079132

Medina, J. (2012). *The epistemology of resistance: Gender and racial oppression, epistemic injustice, and the social imagination.* Oxford: Oxford University Press.

Michener, L., Cook, J., Ahmed, S. M., Yonas, M. A., Coyne-Beasley, T., & Aguilar-Gaxiola, S. (2012). Aligning the goals of community-engaged research: Why and how academic health centers can successfully engage with communities to improve health. *Academic Medicine, 87*, 285–291.

Paphitis, S., & Kelland, L. (2018). In the red: Between research, activism and community development in a menstruation public health intervention. In C. Macleod, J. Marx, P. Mnyaka, & G. Treharne (Eds.), *Palgrave handbook of ethics in critical research.* Palgrave Macmillan.

Pizarro, M. (1998). "Chicana/o Power!" Epistemology and methodology for social justice and empowerment in Chicana/o communities. *Qualitative Studies in Education, 11*(1), 57–80.

Potts, K., & Brown, L. (2005). Becoming an anti-oppressive researcher. In L. A. Brown & S. Strega (Eds.), *Research as resistance: Critical, indigenous and anti-oppressive approaches* (pp. 255–286). Toronto: Canadian Scholars' Press.

van der Reit, M. (2008). Participatory research and the philosophy of social science beyond the moral imperative. *Qualitative Inquiry, 14*(4), 546–565.

Sofolahan-Oladeinde, Y., Mullins, C. D., & Baquet, C. R. (2015). Using community-based participatory research in patient-centered outcomes research to address health disparities in under-represented communities. *Journal of Comparative Effectiveness Research, 4*(5), 515–523.

Sohng, S. (1996). Participatory and community organizing. *Journal of Sociology and Social Welfare, XXIII*(4), 77–97.

Tegegne, T. K., & Sisay, M. M. (2014). Menstrual hygiene management and school absenteeism among female adolescent students in Northeast Ethiopia. *BMC Public Health, 14*, 1118.

Temper, L., & Bene, D. (2016). Transforming knowledge creation for environmental and epistemic justice. *Current Opinion in Environmental Sustainability, 20*, 41–49.

Vaughn, J. G. (2013). *A review of menstruation hygiene management among schoolgirls in sub-Saharan Africa.* Chapel Hill: University of North Carolina.

Index

Note: *Italic* page numbers refer to figures and page numbers followed by "n" denote endnotes.

Printed and bound by CPI Group (UK) Ltd, Croydon, CR0 4YY

18/10/2024

01776250-0013